PEDIATRIC CLINICS
OF NORTH AMERICA

Children's Health and the Environment: Part II

GUEST EDITORS
Jerome A. Paulson, MD, FAAP
Benjamin A. Gitterman, MD, FAAP

April 2007 • Volume 54 • Number 2

SAUNDERS

An Imprint of Elsevier, Inc.
PHILADELPHIA   LONDON   TORONTO   MONTREAL   SYDNEY   TOKYO

W.B. SAUNDERS COMPANY
A Division of Elsevier Inc.

1600 John F. Kennedy Boulevard • Suite 1800 • Philadelphia, Pennsylvania 19103

http://www.theclinics.com

THE PEDIATRIC CLINICS OF NORTH AMERICA
April 2007
Editor: Carla Holloway

Volume 54, Number 2
ISSN 0031-3955
ISBN-13: 978-1-4160-4353-9
ISBN-10: 1-4160-4353-5

The ideas and opinions expressed in *The Pediatric Clinics of North America* do not necessarily reflect those of the Publisher. The Publisher does not assume any responsibility for any injury and/or damage to persons or property arising out of or related to any use of the material contained in this periodical. The reader is advised to check the appropriate medical literature and the product information currently provided by the manufacturer of each drug to be administered to verify the dosage, the method and duration of administration, or contraindications. It is the responsibility of the treating physician or other health care professional, relying on independent experience and knowledge of the patient, to determine drug dosages and the best treatment for the patient. Mention of any product in this issue should not be construed as endorsement by the contributors, editors, or the Publisher of the product or manufacturers' claims.

The Pediatric Clinics of North America (ISSN 0031-3955) is published bi-monthly by Elsevier Inc. 360 Park Avenue South, New York, NY 10010-1710. Months of publication are February, April, June, August, October, and December. Business and Editorial Offices: 1600 John F. Kennedy Blvd., Suite 1800, Philadelphia, PA 19103-2899. Customer Service Office: 6277 Sea Harbor Drive, Orlando, FL 32887-4800. Periodicals postage paid at New York, NY and additional mailing offices. Subscription prices are $138.00 per year (US individuals), $281.00 per year (US institutions), $187.00 per year (Canadian individuals), $367.00 per year (Canadian institutions), $209.00 per year (international individuals), $367.00 per year (international institutions), $72.00 per year (US students), $110.00 per year (Canadian students), and $110.00 per year (foreign students). To receive students/resident rare, orders must be accompanied by name of affiliated institution, date of term, and the signature of program/residency coordinator on institution letterhead. Orders will be billed at individual rate until proof of status is received. Foreign air speed delivery is included in all Clinics subscription prices. All prices are subject to change without notice. POSTMASTER: Send address changes to *The Pediatric Clinics of North America*, Elsevier Periodicals Customer Service, 6277 Sea Harbor Drive, Orlando, FL 32887-4800. **Customer Service: 1-800-654-2452 (US). From outside of the US, call 1-407-345-4000.** E-mail: hhspcs@harcourt.com.

The Pediatric Clinics of North America is also published in Spanish by McGraw-Hill Inter-americana Editores S.A., Mexico City, Mexico; in Portuguese by Riechmann and Affonso Editores, Rua Comandante Coelho 1085, CEP 21250, Rio de Janeiro, Brazil; and in Greek by Althayia SA, Athens, Greece.

The Pediatric Clinics of North America is covered in *Index Medicus, Excerpta Medica, Current Contents, Current Contents/Clinical Medicine, Science Citation Index, ASCA, ISI/BIOMED,* and *BIOSIS.*

Printed in the United States of America.

GUEST EDITORS

JEROME A. PAULSON, MD, FAAP, Associate Professor of Pediatrics and Public Health, Co-Director, Mid-Atlantic Center for Children's Health and the Environment, George Washington University, Washington, District of Columbia

BENJAMIN A. GITTERMAN, MD, FAAP, Associate Professor of Pediatrics and Public Health, Co-Director, Mid-Atlantic Center for Children's Health and the Environment, George Washington University, Washington, District of Columbia

CONTRIBUTORS

MARK E. ANDERSON, MD, Associate Professor of Pediatrics, Denver Health Affiliate, University of Colorado Denver and Health Sciences Center, Denver, Colorado

DAVID C. BELLINGER, PhD, MSc, Professor of Neurology, Harvard Medical School; Professor, Department of Environmental Health, Harvard School of Public Health; and Senior Research Associate in Neurology, Children's Hospital, Boston, Massachusetts

GREGORY M. BOGDAN, PhD, Associate Professor of Pharmaceutical Sciences, Denver Health Affiliate, University of Colorado Denver and Health Sciences Center, Rocky Mountain Poison and Drug Center, Denver, Colorado

IRENA BUKA, MBChB, FRCPC, Associate Clinical Professor of Paediatrics, University of Alberta; and Pediatrician, Misericordia Community Hospital and Health Centre, Edmonton, Alberta, Canada

JACK C. CLIFTON II, MD, MS, Director of Clinical Services, Great Lakes Center for Children's Environmental Health, John H. Stroger, Jr. Hospital of Cook County; Section of Clinical Toxicology and Departments of Internal Medicine, Pediatrics and Pharmacology, Rush University Medical Center; and Toxicon Consortium, Chicago, Illinois

KRISTIE L. EBI, PhD, MPH, ESS, LLC, Alexandria, Virginia

MARION J. FEDORUK, MD, CIH, DABT, Clinical Professor of Medicine, Division of Occupational and Environmental Medicine, University of California, Irvine, School of Medicine; and Center for Occupational & Environmental Health, Irvine, California

ERIC I. FELNER, MD, Director of Pediatric Endocrinology, Hughes Spalding Children's Hospital; and Assistant Professor of Pediatrics, Emory University School of Medicine, Atlanta, Georgia

HOWARD FRUMKIN, MD, DrPH, Director, National Center for Environmental Health/Agency for Toxic Substances and Disease Registry, Centers for Disease Control and Prevention, Atlanta, Georgia

ROBERT J. GELLER, MD, Director, Emory Southeast Pediatric Environmental Health Specialty Unit; Director, Georgia Poison Center; and Associate Professor of Pediatrics, Emory University School of Medicine, Atlanta, Georgia

BENJAMIN A. GITTERMAN, MD, FAAP, Associate Professor of Pediatrics and Public Health, Co-Director, Mid-Atlantic Center for Children's Health and the Environment, George Washington University, Washington, District of Columbia

ROSE GOLDMAN, MD, MPH, Associate Professor of Medicine, Harvard Medical School, Boston; Co-Director, New England Pediatric Environmental Health Subspecialty Unit, Boston; Associate Professor, Department of Environmental Health, Harvard School of Public Health, Boston; and Chief, Director, Division of Occupational & Environmental Medicine, Cambridge Hospital, Cambridge, Massachusetts

TEE L. GUIDOTTI, MD, MPH, DABT, Professor of Occupational and Environmental Medicine; Director, Center for Risk Science and Public Health; and Co-Director, Mid-Atlantic Center for Children's Health and the Environment, School of Public Health and Health Services, George Washington University Medical Center, Washington, District of Columbia

HAROLD E. HOFFMAN, MD, FRCPC, FACOEM, Occupational & Environmental Medicine; and Adjunct Associate Clinical Professor of Occupational Medicine, University of Alberta, Edmonton, Alberta, Canada

BRIAN L. HOLTZCLAW, BS, Environmental Engineer, United States Environmental Protection Agency, Region 4, Atlanta, Georgia

JANICE T. NODVIN, BA, Project Administrator, Emory Southeast Pediatric Environmental Health Specialty Unit; and Institute for the Study of Disadvantage and Disability, Atlanta, Georgia

JEROME A. PAULSON, MD, FAAP, Associate Professor of Pediatrics and Public Health, Co-Director, Mid-Atlantic Center for Children's Health and the Environment, George Washington University, Washington, District of Columbia

SCOTT PHILLIPS, MD, FACP, FACMT, Associate Clinical Professor of Medicine, Division of Clinical Pharmacology & Toxicology, University of Colorado Health Sciences Center, Lone Tree, Colorado

LISA RAGAIN, MAT, Research Associate, Center for Risk Science and Public Health, George Washington University, Washington, District of Columbia

I. LESLIE RUBIN, MD, President, Institute for the Study of Disadvantage and Disability; Co-Director, Emory Southeast Pediatric Environmental Health Specialty Unit; Medical Director, The Team Centers and Developmental Pediatrics Specialists; and Visiting Scholar, Department of Pediatrics, Morehouse School of Medicine, Atlanta, Georgia

JAMES M. SELTZER, MD, Clinical Professor of Medicine, Division of Occupational and Environmental Medicine, University of California, Irvine, School of Medicine, Irvine, California; and Co-Director, Pediatric Environmental Health Specialty Unit, United States Environmental Protection Agency, Region 9, San Francisco, California

W. GERALD TEAGUE, MD, Co-Director, Emory Southeast Pediatric Environmental Health Specialty Unit; and Professor of Pediatrics, Environmental, and Occupational Health, Emory University School of Medicine, Atlanta, Georgia

ALAN D. WOOLF, MD, MPH, Associate Professor of Pediatrics, Harvard Medical School; Co-Director, New England Pediatric Environmental Health Subspecialty Unit; and Staff Pediatrician, Division of General Pediatrics, Children's Hospital, Boston, Massachusetts

CONTENTS

toxicity, infection, and irritation. Some adverse health outcomes have been attributed to mold for which mechanisms of injury are not well defined or are implausible. This article discusses these adverse health outcomes, focusing predominantly on those for which valid associations have been established.

Children are uniquely vulnerable to environmental health problems. Developed countries report as the most common problems ambient (outdoor) air pollution and lead. Developing countries have a wider range of common problems, including childhood injuries, indoor air pollution, infectious disease, and poor sanitation with unsafe water. Globally, the agencies of the United Nations act to protect children and perform essential reporting and standards-setting functions. Conditions vary greatly among countries and are not always better in developing countries. Protecting the health of children requires strengthening the public health and medical systems in every country, rather than a single global agenda.

Children spend much of their waking time at school. Many of the factors in the school environment can be improved with careful planning and allocation of resources. The pediatrician, as a child advocate, is in an excellent position to influence the allocation of school resources to improve the educational outcome. This article summarizes some of the current understanding gathered from applying an environmental health approach to the school setting and provides a basis for the interested physician and other child advocate to learn more and get involved.

The health and well-being of children are critically dependent on the environment in which they live. This article explores the complex relationship between the environment in which a child lives and the environmental factors that can adversely affect health and development. It also examines how awareness of these adverse factors can be helpful in promoting optimal health for children through the societal infrastructures that deal with health, the environment, and social justice.

> Medical laboratory testing is vital for investigating and managing children who have environmentally related disorders and children with environmental chemical exposures. Few of these compounds can be measured in a routine clinical service laboratory. An understanding of the exposure circumstances and toxicology of the agent is required for the ordering and interpretation of tests. Test interpretation requires understanding of the capabilities and limitations of these tests. Adequate investigation, management, and follow-up of exposed children are mandatory.

GOAL STATEMENT

The goal of *Pediatric Clinics of North America* is to keep practicing physicians and residents up to date with current clinical practice in pediatrics by providing timely articles reviewing the state-of-the-art in patient care.

ACCREDITATION

The *Pediatric Clinics of North America* is planned and implemented in accordance with the Essential Areas and Policies of the Accreditation Council for Continuing Medical Education (ACCME) through the joint sponsorship of the University Of Virginia School Of Medicine and Elsevier. The University Of Virginia School of Medicine is accredited by the ACCME to provide continuing medical education for physicians.

The University of Virginia School of Medicine designates this educational activity for a maximum of 15 *AMA PRA Category 1 Credits™*. Physicians should only claim credit commensurate with the extent of their participation in the activity.

The American Medical Association has determined that physicians not licensed in the US who participate in this CME activity are eligible for 15 *AMA PRA Category 1 Credits.™*

Credit can be earned by reading the text material, taking the CME examination online at http://www.theclinics.com/home/cme, and completing the evaluation. After taking the test, you will be required to review any and all incorrect answers. Following completion of the test and evaluation, your credit will be awarded and you may print your certificate.

FACULTY DISCLOSURE/CONFLICT OF INTEREST

The University of Virginia School of Medicine, as an ACCME accredited provider, endorses and strives to comply with the Accreditation Council for Continuing Medical Education (ACCME) Standards of Commercial Support, Commonwealth of Virginia statutes, University of Virginia policies and procedures, and associated federal and private regulations and guidelines on the need for disclosure and monitoring of proprietary and financial interests that may affect the scientific integrity and balance of content delivered in continuing medical education activities under our auspices.

The University of Virginia School of Medicine requires that all CME activities accredited through this institution be developed independently and be scientifically rigorous, balanced and objective in the presentation/discussion of its content, theories and practices.

All authors/editors participating in an accredited CME activity are expected to disclose to the readers relevant financial relationships with commercial entities occurring within the past 12 months (such as grants or research support, employee, consultant, stock holder, member of speakers bureau, etc.). The University of Virginia School of Medicine will employ appropriate mechanisms to resolve potential conflicts of interest to maintain the standards of fair and balanced education to the reader. Questions about specific strategies can be directed to the Office of Continuing Medical Education, University of Virginia School of Medicine, Charlottesville, Virginia.

The authors/editors listed below have identified no financial or professional relationships for themselves or their spouse/partner:
Mark E. Anderson, MD; David Bellinger, PhD, MSc; Gregory M. Bogdan, PhD; Irena Buka, MBChB, FRCPC; Jack Clifton, MD; Kristie L. Ebi, PhD, MPH; M. Joseph Fedoruk, MD, CIH, DABT; Eric Felner, MD; Howard Frumkin, MD, DrPH; Robert J. Geller, MD; Tee L. Guidotti, MD, MPH; Benjamin A. Gitterman, MD (Guest Editor); Rose Goldman, MD, MPH; Harold Hoffman, MD, FRCPC, FACOEM; Carla Holloway (Acquisitions Editor); Brian Holtzclaw; Janice T. Nodvin, BA; Scott Phillips, MD, FACP, FACMT; Lisa Ragain, MAT; I.L. Rubin, MD; James M. Seltzer, MD; W. Gerald Teague, MD; and, Alan D. Woolf, MD, MPH.

The authors/editors listed below identified the following professional or financial affiliations for themselves or their spouse/partner:
Jerome A. Paulson, MD (Guest Editor) owns stock in renal Ventures Ltd, Dialysis.

Disclosure of Discussion of Non-FDA Approved Uses for Pharmaceutical and/or Medical Devices.
The University of Virginia School of Medicine, as an ACCME provider, requires that all authors identify and disclose any "off label" uses for pharmaceutical and medical device products. The University of Virginia School of Medicine recommends that each physician fully review all the available data on new products or procedures prior to clinical use.

TO ENROLL

To enroll in the Pediatric Clinics of North America Continuing Medical Education program, call customer service at 1-800-654-2452 or visit us online at www.theclinics.com/home/cme. The CME program is available to subscribers for an additional fee of $195.00.

FORTHCOMING ISSUES

RECENT ISSUES

ELSEVIER
SAUNDERS

Pediatr Clin N Am
54 (2007) xiii–xiv

PEDIATRIC CLINICS

OF NORTH AMERICA

Preface

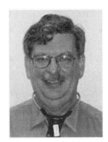 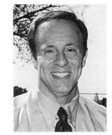

Jerome A. Paulson, MD, FAAP   Benjamin A. Gitterman, MD, FAAP
Guest Editors

Children's environmental health is one of the up-and-coming challenges of the twenty-first century. Palfrey and colleagues [1] have coined the term "millennial morbidities" to describe the most pressing new morbidities of our time—disorders of the bioenvironmental interface, socioeconomic influences on health, health disparities, technological influences on health, overweight and obesity, and mental health issues. In the last century the progress in the treatment of previously identified health care problems in many pediatric subspecialties, although hardly complete, has been spectacular. We now are in an era in which factors that affect the health of children increasingly are identified before the damage is evident, as evidenced by our increasing abilities to identify prenatal and genetically based conditions. Similarly, the impacts of environmental exposures are being understood, and, perhaps more importantly, are being recognized by larger segments of the health professional community and the public alike. Pediatricians now have a responsibility to improve their recognition and understanding of these exposures and to assess and communicate to others the potential risks and threats that environmental exposures pose to children. Finally, this increased understanding underscores the increasing need for pediatricians to be able to act on behalf of children and to do so through increased familiarity with and access to resources that can be of practical benefit to doctors and patients alike.

The *Pediatric Clinics of North America* first published an issue on children's environmental health in 2001. New and increasingly sophisticated information in this field is already available. Expanded resources now exist to

doi:10.1016/j.pcl.2007.02.003   *pediatric.theclinics.com* support child health professionals. The previous publication thoughtfully addressed many of the more obvious and traditional subjects in this field, for the first time in one volume. In this and the previous issue of *Pediatric Clinics of North America*, we offer a collection of articles that address a wider range of environmental health issues that impact children in a number of settings as well as a discussion of issues that the public may be bring to us as health professionals.

At the time of the original publication, the Pediatric Environmental Health Specialty Units were just getting organized. Now a network of 12 units serves all regions of the United States as well as much of North America. Individuals from these units form the core of the group of authors for these issues of *Pediatric Clinics*. The expertise in each of the units individually and in all of the units cumulatively is exceedingly broad and serves as an important resource for education and clinical consultation.

The other articles in this issue of *Pediatric Clinics* are drawn from several of the Centers for Children's Environmental Health and Disease Prevention Research located throughout the country. These centers are the research engine in the nascent but rapidly expanding field of children's health and the environment.

These new collections of articles should be highly relevant to the knowledge and work of medical, nursing, and public health professionals involved in all realms and specialties of pediatric health.

Jerome A. Paulson, MD, FAAP
Associate Professor of Pediatrics and Public Health
Co-Director, Mid-Atlantic Center for Children's Health and the Environment
George Washington University, 2100 M Street NW
Suite 203, Washington, DC 20052, USA

E-mail address: jpaulson@cnmc.org

Benjamin A. Gitterman, MD, FAAP
Associate Professor of Pediatrics and Public Health
Co-Director, Mid-Atlantic Center for Children's Health and the Environment
George Washington University, 2100 M Street NW
Suite 203, Washington, DC 20052, USA

E-mail address: bgitterm@cnmc.org

Reference

[1] Palfrey JS, Tonniges TF, Green M, et al. Introduction: addressing the millennial morbidity—the context of community pediatrics. Pediatrics 2005;115(4 Suppl):1121–3.

ELSEVIER
SAUNDERS

Pediatr Clin N Am
54 (2007) xv

PEDIATRIC CLINICS
OF NORTH AMERICA

Dedication

This issue is dedicated to Gwen Paulson and to Anna, Robert and Sara Gitterman. It also is dedicated to the women and men who work tirelessly to improve the environment for children—those in the Office of Children's Health Protection and the rest of the US Environmental Protection Agency (EPA), as well as the National Center for Environmental Health/Agency for Toxic Substances and Disease Registry (NCEH/ATSDR) along with the rest of the Centers for Disease Control and Prevention (CDC). They are striving to create a healthier, safer future for the children of today and for generations to come.

Jerome A. Paulson, MD, FAAP
Benjamin A. Gitterman, MD, FAAP

doi:10.1016/j.pcl.2007.02.004

ELSEVIER
SAUNDERS

Pediatr Clin N Am
54 (2007) 213–226

PEDIATRIC CLINICS
OF NORTH AMERICA

Climate Change and Children

Kristie L. Ebi, PhD, MPH[a],*, Jerome A. Paulson, MD[b,c,d]

[a]ESS, LLC, 5249 Tancreti Lane, Alexandria, VA 22304, USA
[b]George Washington University School of Medicine and Health Sciences,
2300 I Street NW, Washington, DC 20037, USA
[c]George Washington University School of Public Health and Health Services,
2300 I Street NW, Washington, DC 20037, USA
[d]Mid-Atlantic Center for Children's Health and the Environment,
2300 M Street NW, #203, Washington, DC 20052, USA

The increasing temperatures, changing precipitation patterns, and more extreme weather events that are occurring because of climate change [1] have begun to increase morbidity and mortality from climate-sensitive health determinants and outcomes [2,3]. Children are particularly vulnerable to many of these health outcomes because of their potentially greater exposures (resulting, in part, from behavioral patterns), greater sensitivity to certain exposures, and dependence on caregivers for appropriate preparedness and response. These factors can interact with poverty, race, and class to increase risk further. Because vulnerability to some climate-sensitive health outcomes changes with age, education programs could prepare children for future risks. Consideration of the health impacts of climate change raises issues of intergenerational equity.

Although it should be obvious that children are particularly vulnerable to the changes brought by climate change, little has been written that focuses on the special risks posed to children [4,5]. This article first reviews the key issues related to climate change, then reviews climate-sensitive health determinants and outcomes in the context of children's health, considers intergenerational equity issues, and finishes with a discussion of opportunities for reducing current and projected vulnerabilities to climate change.

Climate change

The earth's climate is determined by complex interactions that involve the sun, oceans, atmosphere, cryosphere (which includes sea ice, freshwater ice,

* Corresponding author.
E-mail address: krisebi@essllc.org (K.L. Ebi).

0031-3955/07/$ - see front matter © 2007 Elsevier Inc. All rights reserved.
doi:10.1016/j.pcl.2007.01.004
pediatric.theclinics.com

snow, glaciers, frozen ground, and permafrost), land surface, and biosphere. These interactions are based on physical laws: conservation of mass, conservation of energy, and Newton's second law of motion. The principal driving force for weather and climate is the uneven warming of the earth's surface because of the tilt in the axis of rotation. In addition to complex and changing atmospheric and oceanic patterns redistributing solar energy from the equator to the poles, some absorbed solar radiation is reradiated as long-wave (infrared) radiation. Some of this infrared radiation is absorbed by the atmospheric greenhouse gases (including water vapor, carbon dioxide [CO_2], methane, nitrous oxide, halocarbons, and ozone) and is reradiated back to the earth, thereby warming the surface more than would be achieved by incoming solar radiation alone and raising the global average surface temperature to its current 15°C (59°F) [6]. Without this warming, the earth's diurnal temperature range would increase dramatically, and the global average surface temperature would be about 33°C (91°F) colder. Although atmospheric concentrations of greenhouse gases have varied over geologic history, they have not been higher than current concentrations for hundreds of thousands, perhaps millions, of years. Based on the physical laws governing climate, increasing concentrations of greenhouse gases will increase the amount of heat in the atmosphere, which will warm the earth further. Fig. 1 illustrates the greenhouse effect.

CO_2 is the most important anthropogenic greenhouse gas. CO_2 is not destroyed chemically; its removal from the atmosphere occurs through multiple processes that store the carbon transiently in land and ocean reservoirs and ultimately in mineral deposits [1]. Natural processes currently remove about half the incremental anthropogenic CO_2 added to the atmosphere annually; the balance is removed over 100 to 200 years [7]. Atmospheric concentrations of CO_2 have increased by 31% since 1750 to about 370 ppm by volume [1]. This concentration has not been exceeded during the past 420,000 years and probably not during the past 20 million years. About 75% of the anthropogenic CO_2 emissions to the atmosphere during the past 20 years resulted from fossil fuel burning; most of the rest resulted from changes in land use, especially deforestation [1].

Instrumental records of temperature, precipitation, and other weather elements began in the 1860s. In its Third Assessment Report, the Intergovernmental Panel on Climate Change (IPCC) evaluated this record and concluded that during the twentieth century, the global average surface temperature increased about 0.6°C ± 0.2°C (1.1°F ± 0.4°F), with the 1990s being the warmest decade [1]. Global surface temperatures increased by about 0.2°C (0.4°F) per decade in the past 30 years [8]. The warmth of the 1990s was outside the 95% confidence interval of temperature uncertainty, defined by historical variation, during even the warmest periods of the last millennium [1]. Further, the IPCC concluded that most of the warming observed during the past 50 years is attributable to human activities, and that human influences will continue to change atmospheric composition throughout the

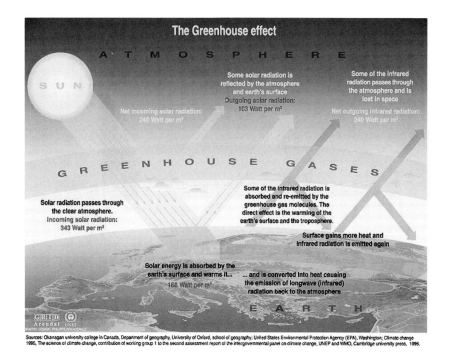

Fig. 1. Greenhouse effect. (*From:* United Nations Environment Programme GRID-Adrenal. Available at: http://www.grida.no/climate/vital/03.htm, Accessed December 20, 2006; with permission).

twenty-first century. The earth is now within about 1°C (1.8°F) of the maximum temperature of the past million years [8].

By 2100, atmospheric concentrations of CO_2 are projected to be between 490 and 1260 ppm (75%–350% above the concentration of 280 ppm in the year 1750) [1]. As a consequence, the global mean surface temperature is projected to increase by between 1.4°C and 5.8°C (2.5°F and 10.4°F) during the same period (Fig. 2). The projected rate of warming is much larger than the observed changes during the twentieth century and is likely to be without precedent during at least the last 10,000 years. The half-life of CO_2 and other greenhouse gases means that the earth is committed to decades of climate change; only beyond mid-century could mitigation efforts begin to reduce projected increases in global mean temperatures [1].

Temperature increases will not be spatially uniform. Average temperature increases are projected to be greatest in the northern regions of North America, Europe, and in northern and central Asia. Precipitation is projected to increase over the northern mid to high latitudes. Climate change also will be characterized by changes in global precipitation patterns, rising sea levels, and increases in the frequency and intensity of some extreme

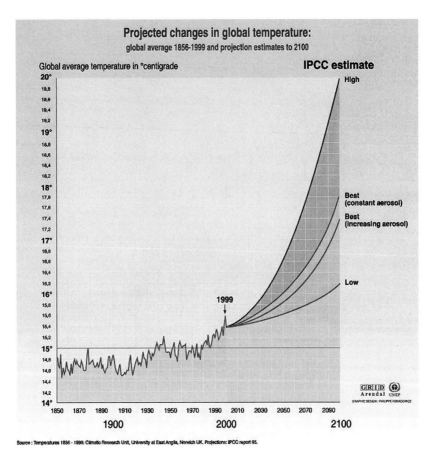

Fig. 2. Projected changes in global average surface temperatures. IPCC, Intergovernmental Panel on Climate Change. (*From:* United Nations Environment Programme GRID-Adrenal. Available at: http://www.grida.no/climate/vital/36.htm, Accessed December 20, 2006; with permission).

weather events. Easterling and colleagues [9] evaluated modeling results of different types of climate extremes for the twenty-first century and concluded that the following changes are likely to occur (90%–99% probability):

Higher maximum temperatures, more hot summer days
An increase in the heat index
More heavy 1-day precipitation events
More heavy multiday precipitation events

It is very likely there will be more frequent and more intense heat waves, and it is possible (33%–66% probability) that there will be more intense mid-latitude storms and more intense El Niño events [9,10].

Climate-sensitive health determinants and outcomes

Weather, climate variability, and climate change can affect children directly and indirectly (Fig. 3). Directly, extreme weather events (such as floods, droughts, and windstorms) and heat events annually affect millions of people and cause billions of dollars of damage. In 2003 in Europe, Canada, and the United States, floods and storms resulted in 101 people dead or missing and caused $9.73 billion in insured damages [11]. More than 35,000 excess deaths were attributed to the extended heat wave in Europe during the same year [12,13]. Indirectly, climate can affect health through changes in the geographic range and intensity of transmission of vector-, tick-, and rodent-borne diseases and food- and waterborne diseases and through changes in the prevalence of diseases associated with air pollutants and aeroallergens. Climate change could alter or disrupt natural systems, making it possible for diseases to spread or emerge in areas where they had been limited or had not existed or for diseases to disappear by making areas less hospitable to the vector or the pathogen [7]. Children in the United States are most likely to be affected by air pollutants and aeroallergens, food- and waterborne diseases, vector-borne diseases, and extreme weather events.

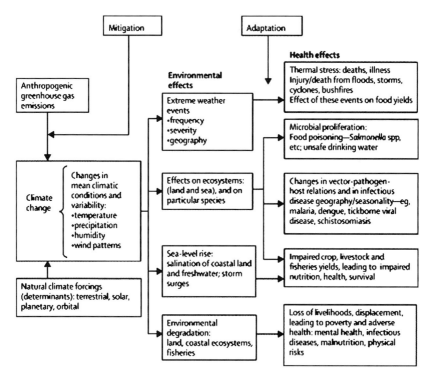

Fig. 3. Schematic summary of main pathways by which climate change affects population health. (*From*: McMichael AJ, Woodruff RE, Hales S. Climate change and human health: present and future risks. Lancet 2006;367:860; with permission.)

The cause-and-effect chain from climate change to changing patterns of health determinants and outcomes is often extremely complex and includes factors such as wealth, distribution of income, status of the public health infrastructure, provision of medical care, and access to adequate nutrition, safe water, and sanitation [14]. Therefore, the severity of future impacts will be determined by changes in climate and by concurrent changes in non-climatic factors and by the adaptation measures implemented to reduce negative impacts.

The potential climate change–related health impacts of extreme weather and temperature events, infectious diseases, and air pollutants are summarized here, followed by a summary of global assessments of current and future disease burdens attributable to climate change.

Extreme weather and heat events

Children are particularly vulnerable in extreme events because of their dependence on adults to ensure their safety and well-being [15]. Because of their size and because of the differences in physiology and psychology, children need specialized medical care during and after man-made and natural disasters [16]. The health and social burden of extreme weather events can be complex, far-reaching, and difficult to attribute to the event itself [17,18]. Adverse health impacts of floods and windstorms include the physical health effects experienced during the event or clean-up process or brought about by damage to infrastructure, including population displacement. Extreme weather events also are associated with mental health effects resulting from the experience of the event or from the recovery process. These psychologic effects tend to be much longer lasting and can be worse than the direct physical effects [17,18].

Heat events affect human health through heat stress, heatstroke, and death [19] as well as exacerbating underlying conditions that can lead to an increase in all-cause mortality [20]. Although heat-related deaths could increase with climate change [21–24], incomplete understanding of how future populations might acclimate to warmer temperatures limits confidence in the size of projected impacts. Regular reports of infants dying when left unintended in vehicles suggest a generally low awareness of the dangers of heat events [25]. In the United States, most deaths associated with heat events have been in older adults [26].

Infectious diseases

Climate and anomalous weather events influence the geographic range and intensity of transmission of several vector-, rodent-, and tick-borne diseases by hindering or enhancing vector and parasite development and survival, including Lyme diseases, St. Louis encephalitis, and West Nile virus. Climate is a primary determinant of whether a particular location has environmental conditions suitable for disease transmission. A change in temperature may lengthen or shorten the season during which vectors or parasites can survive. Small changes in temperature or precipitation may cause previously inhospitable altitudes or ecosystems to become conducive to disease transmission (or cause currently hospitable conditions to become inhospitable). Climate is not the only determinant of vector-borne diseases, however; the many determinants often form an interconnected web with positive feedbacks between transmission dynamics and other factors [27].

Studies have suggested that the changing weather patterns associated with climate change could increase tick populations and the incidence of Lyme disease [28,29]. Hjelle and Glass [30] reported an association between the increased climate variability associated with the El Niño events and rodent-borne outbreaks of Hantavirus. With natural reservoirs in animal populations, the emergence or re-emergence of diseases involves complex interactions [13,30]. Children may be at increased risk for vector-borne diseases because of more time spent outdoors with potentially greater exposure to vectors. For example, in two recent outbreaks, locally caught malaria affected two children in Virginia and one child in Florida [31,32].

A further risk to children (and adults) is the often limited experience of most physicians with emerging and re-emerging diseases. Vectors for dengue fever, malaria, and other diseases are present in many regions of the United States, so there are constant risks for reintroduction of these diseases, particularly with increased international travel. Further, vectors may alter their ranges with changes in temperature and precipitation (see, for example, [29]). After vector control, only prompt diagnosis and treatment can break chains of transmission, suggesting a need for a greater emphasis in medical schools on identification and treatment of these diseases.

Several food- and waterborne diseases are climate sensitive, suggesting the risk of diarrheal illnesses is likely to increase with higher ambient temperatures. An estimated 76 million cases of food-borne disease occur annually in the United States, with 325,000 hospitalizations and 5000 deaths [33]. Common forms of food poisoning such as salmonellosis have an approximately linear association with ambient temperature (see, for example, Refs. [34–36]). Curriero and colleagues [37] and Kistemann and colleagues [38] found that extreme precipitation events increase the loading of contaminants in waterways, and Casman and colleagues [39] concluded that climate change could increase the risk of illness associated with *Cryptosporidium parvum*.

Air pollutants and aeroallergens

There is extensive literature documenting the adverse health impacts of exposure to elevated concentrations of air pollution, especially particulates with aerodynamic diameters under 10 and 2.5 μm, and the air pollutants ozone, sulfur dioxide, nitrogen dioxide, and carbon monoxide. Air pollution concentrations are the result of interactions among local weather patterns, atmospheric circulation features, wind, topography, human responses to weather changes (ie, the onset of cold or warm spells may increase heating and cooling needs and, therefore, an increase in electricity generation), and other factors. Climate change could affect local and regional air quality directly through changes in chemical reaction rates, boundary-layer heights that affect vertical mixing of pollutants, and changes in synoptic airflow patterns that govern pollutant transport [1]. Indirect effects could result from increased or decreased anthropogenic emissions brought about by changes in human behavior or from altered levels of biogenic emissions brought about by higher temperatures and land cover change. Establishing the scale (local, regional, global) and direction of change (improvement or deterioration) of air quality is challenging, however [40].

More is known about the potential impact of climate change on ground-level ozone than on other air pollutants. Changes in concentrations of ground-level ozone driven by scenarios of future emissions and/or weather patterns have been projected for Europe and North America [41–45]. Future emissions are, of course, uncertain and depend on assumptions about population growth, economic development, and energy use [46,47]. In the United States a study of the projected increased adverse health impacts of ozone due to climate change concluded that summer ozone-related mortality could increase by 4% in the New York area by the 2050s based on climatic changes alone [48].

Recent studies examined the potential impact of climate variability and change on airborne allergen concentrations and reached conclusions similar to those of Bernard and colleagues [40]: that increased CO_2 and higher temperatures generally increase the growth rate of allergen-producing plants (eg, ragweed) and the production of pollen [49,50]. D'Amato and colleagues [51] also concluded that air pollution might facilitate the penetration and the depth of penetration of allergens into the lungs, thus increasing the risk of these allergens.

Global assessments of the health impacts of climate change

The most comprehensive evaluation of the burden of disease resulting from climate change used a comparative risk assessment approach as part of the Global Burden of Disease study to project the total health burden attributed to climate change between 2000 and 2030 and to project how much of this burden could be avoided by stabilizing greenhouse gas emissions [2]. Health outcomes were analyzed by region to understand better where current and projected future disease burdens are highest and to identify the outcomes that contribute to the largest share of the total burden. The health outcomes included in the analysis were chosen based on sensitivity to climate variation, likely future importance, and availability of quantitative global models (or feasibility of constructing them) [2]. Specific health out-comes included were episodes of diarrheal disease, cases of *Plasmodium falciparum* malaria, fatal unintentional injuries in coastal floods and inland floods/landslides, and nonavailability of recommended daily calorie intake (as an indicator for the prevalence of malnutrition). In the year 2000, climate change was estimated to have caused the loss of more than 150,000 lives (0.3% of worldwide deaths) and 5,500,000 disability-adjusted life years (0.4% worldwide), with malnutrition accounting for approximately 50% of these deaths and disability-adjusted life years [2,3]. These estimates relate to a period when limited climate change had occurred, suggesting that future studies may find larger health burdens caused by climate change.

The projected relative risks attributable to climate change in 2030 vary by health outcome and region and are largely negative, with the majority of the projected disease burden resulting from increases in diarrheal disease and malnutrition, primarily in low-income populations already experiencing a large burden of disease [2]. Absolute disease burdens depend on assumptions of population growth, future baseline disease incidence, and the extent of adaptation.

Hitz and Smith [52] reviewed the literature on the projected health impacts of climate change and concluded that health risks are more likely to increase than decrease with increasing global mean surface temperature, particularly in low-latitude countries. In addition to greater vulnerability to climate, these countries have some of the largest populations, tend to be less developed, and generally have poorer public health infrastructure, likely leading to greater damages.

Exposure to UV radiation

Climate change has the potential to affect exposure to UV radiation either through its effects on the rate of healing of the stratospheric ozone hole or through its effect on clouds and smog [1]. Climate change is projected to slow the rate of healing of the stratospheric ozone hole, increasing exposure to UV. There are three segments of the UV spectrum, UVA (400–315 nm), UVB (315–280 nm), and UVC (<280 nm). UV exposure, particularly UVB, has potential beneficial and adverse health effects [53,54]. Vitamin D, which is produced by the skin as a result of UV exposure, increases calcium absorption and may protect against various cancers and myocardial infarction and reduce blood pressure. UV exposure also is associated with sunburn, photoaging, the development of cataracts, and the development of basal cell and squamous cell carcinomas and malignant melanoma. Adolescence seems to be a critical period for increased risk of development of subsequent squamous cell carcinoma and malignant melanoma. UV exposure also down-regulates the immune system in experimental animals; this phenomenon may be part of the causal chain leading to cancer development.

Intergenerational equity

The inherent inertia in the climate system means that the earth is commit-ted to decades of climate change from the greenhouse gases currently in the atmosphere. Even if all greenhouse gas emissions stopped tomorrow, the earth probably will warm 0.5°C to 1.0°C during the next several decades; this warming will be in addition to the 0.6°C increase in global average sur-face temperature that occurred during the last century [1]. This probability raises intergenerational equity issues: the actions (or lack thereof) taken today will affect not only the climate for present adults' children and grand-children, but also the costs of actions taken to adapt to and mitigate climate change [55]. Actions taken in the next 10 to 20 years will have only a limited effect on the climate over the next 40 to 50 years, but investing in mitigation now may avoid some of the severe consequences projected for later in the century. The longer serious reductions in greenhouse gas emissions are delayed, the higher will be the projected costs for both mitigation and adap-tation, with these costs borne by future generations. Another intergenera-tional equity issue is that some impacts of climate change, such as the rise in sea level inundating low-lying coastal areas and some small island states, cannot be avoided. The unavoidable impacts will increase with increasing atmospheric concentrations of greenhouse gases.

Because fossil fuel combustion is a source of urban air pollutants and greenhouse gases, policies to reduce greenhouse gas emissions can have health benefits in the near and long term for children and adults. For exam-ple, there are potential synergies in reducing greenhouse gases and improv-ing population health by creating sustainable transport systems that make more use of public transport, walking, and cycling [56]. For other energy sources, health-impact assessments should be conducted to evaluate positive and negative health impacts.

**Opportunities for reducing current and future vulnerabilities
to climate change**

Climate change will make more difficult the control of climate-sensitive health determinants and outcomes. Therefore, health policies need explicitly to incorporate climate-related risks to maintain current levels of control [57]. In most cases, the primary response will be to enhance current health risk management activities. The health determinants and outcomes that are pro-jected to increase with climate change are problems today (by definition, new risks are problematic to project). In some cases, programs will need to be implemented in new regions; in others, climate change may reduce cur-rent infectious disease burdens. The degree to which programs and measures will need to be augmented to address the additional pressures caused by cli-mate change will depend on factors such as [57]

The current burden of climate-sensitive diseases
The effectiveness of current interventions
Projections of where, when, and how the burden of disease could change
  with changes in climate and climate variability
The feasibility of implementing additional cost-effective interventions
Other stressors that could increase or decrease resilience to impacts
The social, economic, and political context within which interventions are
  implemented

Although there are uncertainties about future climate change, failure to invest in adaptation may leave communities and nations poorly prepared and increase the probability of severe adverse consequences [56]. Adaptation policies and measures need to consider how effectively and efficiently to reduce climate-related risks within the context of projected demographic, economic, institutional, technologic, and other changes. The current burden of climate-sensitive diseases suggests that adaptation and mitigation policies and measures need to be implemented soon to avoid projected risks caused by climate change.

References

[1] Albritton DL, Meira Filho LG, Cubasch U, et al. Intergovernmental Panel on climate change. Technical summary. Working Group 1: the scientific basis. Cambridge (UK): Cambridge University Press; 2001.
[2] McMichael AJ, Campbell-Lendrum D, Kovats S, et al. Global climate change. In: Ezzati M, Lopez A, Rodgers A, et al, editors. Comparative quantification of health risks: global and regional burden of disease due to selected major risk factors. Geneva (Switerland): World Health Organization; 2004. p. 1543–649.
[3] Patz JA, Campbell-Lendrum D, Holloway T, et al. Impact of regional climate change on human health. Nature 2005;438:310–7.
[4] Bunyavanich S, Landrigan CP, McMichael AJ, et al. The impact of climate change on child health. Ambul Pediatr 2003;3:44–52.
[5] Canadian Institute of Child Health. Changing habits, changing climate. A foundation analysis. 2001. Available at: http://www.cich.ca/PDFFiles/ClimateChangeReport.pdf. Accessed December 23, 2006.
[6] Burroughs WJ. Changing weather. In: Burroughs WJ, editor. Weather. Sudney. The Nature Company Guides/Time-Life Books; 1996.
[7] National Research Council. National Academy of Sciences, Division of Earth and Life Sciences Studies Board on Atmospheric Sciences and Climate Committee on Climate, Ecosystems, Infectious Disease, and Human Health. Under the weather: climate, ecosystems, and infectious disease. Washington, DC: National Academy Press; 2001.
[8] Hansen J, Sato M, Ruedy R, et al. Global temperature change. Proc Natl Acad Sci U S A 2006;103:14288–93.
[9] Easterling DR, Evans JL, Groisman PY, et al. Observed variability and trends in extreme climate events. Bulletin of the American Meteorological Society 2000;81:417–25.
[10] Meehl G, Tebaldi C. More intense, more frequent and longer lasting heat waves in the 21st century. Nature 2004;305:994–7.
[11] Natural catastrophes and man-made disasters in 2003. Zurich: Swiss Re. 2004 Sigma 1/2004.

[12] Kosatsky T. The 2003 European heat waves. Euro Surveill 2005;10:148–9.
[13] McMichael A, Githeko A, Akhtar R, et al. In: McCarthy JJ, Canziani OF, Leary N, et al, editors. Human population health. Climate change 2001. Impacts, adaptations and vulnerability. Contribution of Working Group II to the third assessment report of the Intergovernmental Panel on Climate Change. New York: Cambridge University Press; 2001. p. 453–85.
[14] Woodward A, Hales S, Weinstein P. Climate change and human health in the Asia Pacific region: who will be the most vulnerable? Climate Research 1998;11:31–7.
[15] Shapiro A, Seim L, Christensen RC, et al. Chronicles from out-of-state professionals: providing primary care to underserved children after a disaster: a national organization response. Pediatrics 2006;117:S412–41.
[16] Weiner DL, Manzi SF, Waltzman ML, et al. FEMA's organized response with a pediatric subspecialty team: the National Disaster Medical System: a pediatric perspective. Pediatrics 2006;117:S405–11.
[17] Ahern MJ, Kovats RS, Wilkinson P, et al. Global health impacts of floods: epidemiological evidence. Epidemiol Rev 2005;27:36–45.
[18] Hajat S, Ebi K, Kovats S, et al. The human health consequences of flooding in Europe and the implications for public health: a review of the evidence. Applied Environmental Science and Public Health 2003;1:13–21.
[19] Kilbourne EM. Heat waves and hot environments. In: Noji EK, editor. The public health consequences of disasters. New York: Oxford University Press; 1997. p. 245–69.
[20] Kovats RS, Koppe C. Heat waves: past and future impacts. In: Ebi KL, Smith JB, Burton I, editors. Integration of public health with adaptation to climate change: lessons learned and new directions. London: Taylor & Francis; 2005. p. 136–60.
[21] Dessai S. Heat stress and mortality in Lisbon part II. An assessment of the potential impacts of climate change. Int J Biometeorol 2003;48:37–44.
[22] Hayhoe K, Cayan D, Field CB, et al. Emission pathways, climate change, and impacts on California. Proc Natl Acad Sci U S A 2004;101:12422–7.
[23] Keatinge WR, Donaldson GC, Kovats RS, et al. Heat and cold related mortality morbidity and climate change. In: Health effects of climate change in the UK. London: Department of Health; 2002. p. 70–80.
[24] McMichael A, Woodruff R, Whetton P, et al. Human health and climate change in Oceania: risk assessment 2002. Canberra (Australia): Commonwealth of Australia; 2003.
[25] Guard A, Gallagher SS. Heat related deaths in young children in parked cars: an analysis of 171 fatalities in the United States, 1995–2002. Inj Prev 2005;11:33–7.
[26] Centers for Disease Control and Prevention (CDC). Heat-related deaths—Chicago, Illinois, 1996–2001, and United States, 1979–1999. MMWR Morb Mortal Wkly Rep 2003; 52:610–3.
[27] Chan NY, Smith F, Wilson TF, et al. An integrated assessment framework for climate change and infectious diseases. Environ Health Perspect 1999;107:329–37.
[28] Subak S. Effects of climate on variability in Lyme disease Incidence in northeastern United States. Am J Epidemiol 2003;157:531–8.
[29] Ogden NH, Maarouf A, Barker IK, et al. Climate change and the potential for range expansion of the Lyme disease vector Ixodes scapularis in Canada. Int J Parasitol 2006; 36:63–70.
[30] Hjelle B, Glass GE. Outbreak of hantavirus infection in the Four Corners region of the United States in the wake of the 1997–1998 El Nino-southern oscillation. J Infect Dis 2000;181:1569–73.
[31] Centers for Disease Control and Prevention. Local transmission of Plasmodium vivax malaria –Virginia. MMWR Morb Mortal Wkly Rep 2002;51:921–3.
[32] Centers for Disease Control and Prevention. Local transmission of Plasmodium vivax malaria—Palm Beach County, Florida, 2003. MMWR Morb Mortal Wkly Rep 2006;55: 908–11.

[33] Centers for Disease Control and Prevention. 2006. The foodnet program of the CDC. Available at: http://www.cdc.gov/ncidod/dbmd/diseaseinfo/foodborneinfections_g.htm. Accessed October 31, 2006.

[34] D'Souza RM, Becker NG, Hall G, et al. Does ambient temperature affect foodborne disease? Epidemiology 2004;15:86–92.

[35] Fleury M, Charron D, Holt J, et al. A time series analysis of the relationship of ambient temperature and common bacterial enteric infections in to Canadian provinces. Int J Biometeorol 2006;50:385–91.

[36] Kovats RS, Edwards SJ, Hajat S, et al. The effect of temperature on food poisoning: a time-series analysis of salmonellosis in ten European countries. Epidemiol Infect 2004;132: 443–53.

[37] Curriero FC, Patz JA, Rose JB, et al. The association between extreme precipitation and waterborne disease outbreaks in the United States, 1948–1994. Am J Public Health 2001; 91:1172–4.

[38] Kistemann T, Claben T, Koch C, et al. Microbial load of drinking water reservoir tributaries during extreme rainfall and runoff. App Environ Microbiol 2002;68:2188–97.

[39] Casman EA, Fischhoff B, Palmgren C, et al. An integrated risk model of a drinking water-borne cryptosporidiosis outbreak. Risk Anal 2000;20:495–511.

[40] Bernard SM, Samet JM, Grambsch A, et al. The potential impacts of climate variability and change on air pollution-related health effects in the United States. Environ Health Perspect 2001;109(Suppl 2):199–209.

[41] Derwent RG, Collins WJ, Johnson CE, et al. Transient behaviour of tropospheric ozone precursors in a global 3-D CTM and their indirect greenhouse effects. Clim Change 2001;49: 463–87.

[42] Hogrefe C, Biswas J, Lynn B, et al. Simulating regional-scale ozone climatology over the eastern United States: model evaluation results. Atmos Environ 2004;38:2627.

[43] Johnson CS, Stevenson DS, Collins W, et al. Role of climate feedback on methane and ozone studied with a coupled ocean-atmosphere-chemistry model. Geophys Res Lett 2001;28: 1723–6.

[44] Stevenson DS, Johnson CE, Collins WJ, et al. Future estimates of tropospheric ozone radiative forcing and methane turnover—the impact of climate change. Geophys Res Lett 2000; 27:2073–6.

[45] Taha H. Potential impacts of climate change on troposphereic ozone in California: a preliminary episodic modeling assessment of the Los Angeles basin and the Sacramento Valley. Berkeley (CA): Lawrence Berkeley National Laboratories; 2001.

[46] Syri S, Karvosenoja N, Lehtila A, et al. Modeling the impacts of the Finnish climate strategy on air pollution. Atmos Environ 2002;36:3059–69.

[47] Webster M, Babiker M, Mayer M, et al. Uncertainty in emissions projections for climate models. Atmos Environ 2002;36:3659–70.

[48] Knowlton K, Rosenthal JE, Hogrefe C, et al. Assessing ozone-related health impacts under a changing climate. Environ Health Perspect 2004;112:1557–63.

[49] Ziska LH, Gebhard DE, Frenz DA, et al. Cities as harbingers of climate change: ragweed, urbanization, and public health. J Allergy Clin Immunol 2003;111:290–5.

[50] Ziska LH. Evaluation of the growth response of six invasive species to past, present, and future atmospheric carbon dioxide. J Exp Bot 2003;54:395–404.

[51] D'Amato G, Liccardi G, D'Amato M, et al. The role of outdoor air pollution and climatic changes on the rising trends in respiratory allergy. Respir Med 2001;95:606–11.

[52] Hitz S, Smith J. Estimating global impacts from climate change. Glob Environ Change 2004; 14:201–18.

[53] Diffey B. Climate change, ozone depletion and the impact of ultraviolet exposure of human skin. Phys Med Biol 2004;49:R1–11.

[54] Schwarz T. Photoimmunosuppression. Photodermatol Photoimmunol Photomed 2002;18: 141–5.

[55] Stern N. The economics of climate change: The Stern Review; 2007. London: Cabinet Office, HM Treasury; 2007.
[56] Haines A, Kovats RS, Campbell-Lendrum D, et al. Climate change and human health: impacts, vulnerability, and public health. Lancet 2006;367:1–9.
[57] Ebi KL, Smith J, Burton I, et al. Some lessons learned from public health on the process of adaptation. Mitigation and Adaptation Strategies for Global Change 2006;11:601–20.

ELSEVIER
SAUNDERS

Pediatr Clin N Am
54 (2007) 227–235

PEDIATRIC CLINICS
OF NORTH AMERICA

Protecting Children from Toxic Exposure: Three Strategies

Tee L. Guidotti, MD, MPH, DABT[a,b,*], Lisa Ragain, MAT[a]

[a]Center for Risk Science and Public Health, Department of Environmental
and Occupational Health, School of Public Health and Health Services,
George Washington University, Washington, DC, USA
[b]Mid-Atlantic Center for Children's Health and the Environment,
Washington, DC, USA

The terminology used in health protection has a shaping effect on the strategies that can be visualized. The vocabulary used to describe a problem may constrain the imagination of its solution and reflect limitations on conceptualizing the problem. The characterization of the effects a toxic exposure as "poisoning" or as "toxicity" has implications for which intervention strategy makes sense: clinical screening, high-risk hazard control, or all-source reduction of exposure. To a toxicologist, "poisonings" are cases in which the child has a defined pattern of symptoms corresponding to toxic effects at a mid- to high level of exposure. "Toxicity" refers to a broader spectrum of effects, and at the lower levels of exposure the child may have no specific, individual symptoms but still may be affected subclinically. At low levels of exposure, toxic chemicals may act as risk factors in the epidemiologic sense of increasing the probability of a given outcome without being the single determinant cause.

For example, cigarette smoking is a direct cause of some diseases, such as lung cancer and emphysema. It would be meaningful in some contexts to speak of "cigarette poisoning," and occasionally the term is heard

---

The authors have been members of the Lead Elimination Task Force in Washington, DC, and, through George Washington University's Center for Risk Science and Public Health, were retained as consultants in advising the District of Columbia Water and Sewer Authority on risk management during the elevation of lead in drinking water in the city in 2003–2004.

* Corresponding author. Mid-Atlantic Center for Child Health and Environment, George Washington University Medical Center, 2100 M Street, NW, Suite 203, Washington, DC 20052.

E-mail address: eohtlg@gwumc.edu (T.L. Guidotti).

rhetorically. Cigarette smoking, however, is also a risk factor for other out-comes, such as heart disease. In that sense, a toxic effect of cigarette smoke is one among several factors important in the frequency of disease. If the prob-lem of cigarette smoking is taken as one of acute or chronic fatal poisoning, there are arguments for emphasizing smoking cessation in people who have trouble controlling their tobacco habit and therefore reducing the probabil-ity of extreme effects. If the problem is defined as one of preventing chronic "poisoning," development of a "safe" cigarette to reduce the dose and there-fore the probability of symptomatic "poisoning" makes sense for people who cannot quit. If it is defined as a problem of toxicity along a wide spec-trum of effects, discouraging people from putting any combustion product in their mouths is a better strategy. Ideally, all three strategies and all avail-able modalities would be used in contingent fashion, but in practice that never happens. Agencies or smoking cessation programs use one or a limited number of modalities, because the cost of running programs using all avail-able possibilities is too great. For adults, the strategy offered depends in large part on whether the sponsoring agency or the smoker views the problem as a high-risk poisoning with a certain adverse outcome or as a lower-level toxicity that increases the risk of common diseases. This anal-ogy is imperfect but serves to illustrate the concept.

The importance of making a distinction between degrees of poisoning and levels of toxicity is illustrated by lead. Control of lead exposure, like other hazards in developed countries, has reduced the frequency of obvious poisonings, but the problem of low levels of toxicity remains. The spectrum of lead toxicity now is known to include more subtle behavioral and neuro-developmental effects, demonstrable on a population basis, which heavily overlap the normal distribution of ability. Lead exposure in this range there-fore assumes the characteristics of a risk factor rather than a determinant cause. The strategies for prevention are different.

Poisoning versus toxicity

The difference between poisoning and toxicity is not merely semantic or stylistic. The meanings define concepts that, as will be shown, imply different prevention strategies.

To a toxicologist, the word "poisoning" means the presence of symptoms. Toxicology journals tend to be consistent in preferring the term "toxicity" [1]. Usually there is a constellation of symptoms, called a "toxidrome," that, if not unique, is characteristic for a certain toxic exposure. There are many defini-tions of poison but relatively few formal definitions of poisoning. An early for-mal definition of "poisoning" was "the evil effects of any substance," referring to clinical symptoms [2]. Although, unlike the word "poison," which usually is defined on the first page of textbooks, the word "poisoning" often goes unde-fined in the literature of toxicology, but its usage almost always implies visible symptoms and in lay language often implies death. The glossary for the environmental health section of *Healthy People 2010*, for example, provides the following definition for the public: "Poisoning: An exposure to a toxic substance that produces negative signs or symptoms" [3].

Toxicity, on the other hand, is a subtler concept that represents the potential, real or unexpressed, for injury across the entire spectrum of effects. *Stedman's Medical Dictionary* defines "toxicity" as the "quality of being poisonous, especially to the degree of virulence of a toxic microbe or of a poison" [4]. To a toxicologist, toxicity ranges from the earliest subclinical effects inducing an adaptive response to fatality. Textbooks on toxicology consistently use the terms "lead toxicity" when referring to the effects of lead [5–8]. The National Institute of Environmental Health Sciences uses the terms "poison" and "toxicity" differently in their fact sheet on lead: the section "What Is Lead Poisoning?" refers to symptomatic lead toxicity, and "What Is Lead Toxicity?" refers to relatively lower levels of exposure to lead in the body when a child's brain is developing [9].

This usage is not restricted to toxicologists. The US Centers for Disease Control and Prevention (CDC) avoids the term "lead poisoning" in everything but the name of its Lead Poisoning Prevention program. Although the blood lead level of concern is given as 10 µg/dL throughout the text, it is not used explicitly to define lead poisoning, and no specific definition of lead poisoning is given in the text [10]. The CDC's most recent and authoritative document, "Lead Poisoning Prevention in Young Children" (2005) [10] explicitly states that " 'lead poisoning' is generally understood for clinical purposes to refer to episodic, acute, symptomatic illness from lead toxicity" and uses the term only for that meaning and in historical references. The CDC regularly produces a surveillance report in the *Morbidity and Mortality Weekly Report* (*MMWR*) on blood lead levels in the United States, but the surveillance reports do not use the term "lead poisoning" [11]. The text refers to "high blood lead levels." *MMWR* does use the terminology "lead poisoning" with an implicit definition in specific case reports where there are signs and symptoms [12]. Likewise, the Agency for Toxic Substances and Disease Registry, which produces authoritative toxicologic profiles for hazardous substances, does not use the term "lead poisoning" in the toxicological profile for lead. Rather it uses the terms "exposure" and "toxicity," which are described in detail [13]. The American Academy of Pediatrics Clinical Guidelines for Lead Exposure in Children consistently uses the term "elevated blood lead levels" and avoids the phrase "lead poisoning" [14].

Not every source follows the convention of distinguishing poisoning from other forms of toxicity. A fact sheet from Region 2 of the Environmental Protection Agency states, under the heading "What Is Lead Poisoning?" that "lead is a metal that can make infants and young children ill. Many of those affected never even look sick. Sometimes children with lead poisoning can have learning disabilities and other health problems" [15]. This usage equates the spectrum of toxicity, including symptomatic illness, with poisoning but it is an exception in the technical literature.

Public education and outreach programs and public health-oriented agencies seem to prefer the term "lead poisoning." The National Coalition to End Childhood Lead Poisoning has its definition of lead poisoning in the realm of public information: "Lead poisoning occurs when the amount of lead in a person's bloodstream is too high" [16]. The National Safety Council has in-depth information on lead in their public literature. Unique to this organization is the glossary of terms related to childhood lead exposure, including, "Lead poisoning: The level of lead in an individual's blood at which the CDC states that adverse health effects are bound to occur" [17]. This usage is not consistent with CDC's own definitions. The term "toxicity" is not given in this glossary, and the definition of poisoning obviously does not require symptoms.

Implications for lead

Nowhere is this semantic distinction more important than in preventing lead toxicity.

The terms "lead toxicity" and "lead poisoning" tend to be used interchangeably in pediatric practice and public health. This usage is understood to be in part rhetorical and in part philosophical, because the word "poisoning" communicates a sense of urgency, and any degree of avoidable toxicity is unacceptable. It is useful to keep the concepts straight, however, because the meanings are subtly but importantly different, and "toxicity" is the more general term.

Lead poisoning, in the classic, syndromic sense, is now rare. Cardinal symptoms of pediatric lead toxicity include acute encephalopathy, colicky abdominal pain, projectile vomiting, ataxia, and a combination of irritability and lethargy. Such cases have a poor prognosis for full recovery because they are associated with long-term, symptomatic neurologic impairment. Lead poisoning in the classic sense, as used by toxicologists, is controlled by removing sources of exposure that result in symptomatic disease. This approach implies a strategy based on identifying and removing the sources of catastrophic toxicity. Paradoxically, this approach may not do much to reduce mean lead levels in a population.

Historically, the main sources of lead exposure for children in the United States were interior leaded paint, emissions from leaded gasoline, and, in some places, residual lead from primary or secondary smelting activity. The ban on interior leaded paint in 1978 led to a sudden and marked reduction in cases of symptomatic lead poisoning in the United States [18] that has continued to the present day. The residue of lead paint in older housing continues to be a threat to many children, however, especially in cities with older housing stock, such as Washington, DC. The most important sources of lead today are lead paint and, occasionally, lead-contaminated toys. Some consumer products still may contain lead (eg, low-temperature glazed pottery, Ayurvedic medicines, kohl [the South Asian cosmetic], and certain plastic products in which lead is used as a stabilizer), and lead may, rarely, be present in the ink on labels for food products (recently a problem with imported candies). Each of these sources may place the child at risk for acute or chronic, symptomatic toxicity—the condition toxicologists recognize as poisoning. They result in sporadic cases of often severe disease in a relatively small number of children. Removing these sources of lead may reduce the frequency of lead poisoning cases but may have little effect on mean lead levels for the population or the risk of low-level lead toxicity in most children.

Mean blood lead levels in the United States were much higher in previous generations and continue to fall for all ages. Today, the "average" (actually, the geometric mean) blood lead level for American children is about 2 μg/dL [19], probably the lowest it has been for a century, at least in urban areas [18]. This drop in blood lead level may have unmasked relationships between blood lead and low-level toxicity that were not obvious before. For this reason, there has been increasing concern in recent years about the toxicity of lead at lower exposures and about lead as a risk factor for child health and development [20].

Other environmental sources of exposure to lead, such as the persistent residue from leaded gasoline, contribute to high lead levels in dust in homes, which is a major contributor to elevated blood lead levels. The ban on leaded gasoline in 1986 resulted in a rapid and steady decline in the average blood lead level in children, increased the margin of safety, and therefore reduced the likelihood of acute poisoning [18]. The residue of lead in soil contributes to background exposure in urban areas, however, and therefore contributes to body burden and mean lead level. Other secondary sources include food, drinking water, and soil. These sources are highly unlikely to result in lead poisoning, in the classic toxicologic sense, but may contribute to the elevation of blood lead and total body burden. Removing these sources of lead may reduce mean lead levels but probably will do little or nothing to reduce the frequency of symptomatic lead poisoning where it remains a problem.

The CDC has established the "level of concern" for children at 10 μg/dL; all children should be below this level, especially at the critical age of 2 years. Most experts, however, now believe that this level of concern is too low because evidence for neurodevelopmental effects, in the form of group differences in IQ and academic achievement and a higher probability of behavioral abnormalities (including aggression), have been demonstrated even below this level [20–24]. The effects are proportional to blood lead levels and show no evidence for a threshold, suggesting that the lower the lead level is, the better [25]. These are group effects: it is not possible to establish an effect for a particular child. Indeed, for the individual child, an effect associated with lead exposure cannot be discerned; the individual child may fall within the normal range. For this reason, the toxicologist normally would not use the word "poisoning" and would prefer the word "toxicity" because the effect is in the range of toxic effects but also may be within normal limits.

At lower levels of toxicity, exposure to a toxin may be one factor among many in a multifactorial model and may not necessarily be the most powerful risk factor. At ambient environmental levels, exposures to such hazards, including lead, cease to become threats in the toxicologic sense or etiologic causes in the clinical sense and become instead risk factors in the epidemiologic sense, one of many determinants. For example, in the case of subclinical neurotoxicity resulting in learning and behavioral effects, lower-level lead exposure may be one among many environmental determinants, including mercury, arsenic, endocrine disruptors (thyroid hormone mimics), inadequate omega fatty acid intake, inadequate early child stimulation, and a myriad of other influences on early childhood development [26]. Sorting through these various risk factors to ascertain which are most important and which have relatively small effects is the work of epidemiology informed by toxicology. At present, however, it is not possible to estimate attributable risks reliably [27].

Three general protective strategies

There are three basic strategies to protect children: individual intervention, the preventive medicine strategy, and the public health strategy. The latter two are defined here as they were by epidemiologist Rose [28], who developed the concepts with cardiovascular disease in mind.

The first strategy is the individual approach, focused on the individual child. Applied to lead, the individual approach is a lead-poisoning prevention and mitigation strategy. The individual child must be protected by the parent or guardian, family, and immediate community; the basic strategy is through education. Most pediatricians do not have time to educate the parents themselves and so depend on public health–oriented agencies and patient education materials. Protection must be undertaken within the family and focused on identifying and eliminating the specific sources of exposure that the child may encounter. Because neither pediatrician nor public health agency can be omnipresent, the first line of protection is the parent or guardian. To prevent lead poisoning, children are individually protected in or removed from homes where a hazard exists, on a case-by-case basis, but placing such responsibility on the parent is not reliable. The pediatrician may suspect a problem, and an elevated blood lead level confirm the suspicion, but if the child is symptomatic much damage has already been done. In this situation, it may be possible to prevent future disability resulting from further exposure ("tertiary prevention," in the language of public health), but it is too late to prevent the initial injury from past exposure ("primary prevention") [29,30].

The preventive medicine model is based on identifying individuals at high risk and then intervening one-on-one. Applied to lead, this is primarily a lead-poisoning prevention strategy that also reduces the risk of lead toxicity at lower levels, reducing its role as a risk factor for subclinical manifestations in children with slightly or nearly elevated blood lead levels. Identification necessarily requires a screening step, which in the case of lead toxicity is the routine blood lead level. Children in circumstances at high risk for symptomatic poisoning must be screened to be identified, and this information is conveyed to a system that then provides an intervention at the level of the individual child, usually mitigation of exposure to lead paint in the home. When the blood lead level is slightly rather than highly elevated, there is both the risk associated with lower-level toxicity and an increased risk of symptomatic poisoning, because the margin of safety for symptomatic poisoning is reduced (ie, less additional lead intake would be required to push the blood level into a range associated with higher levels of toxicity). Poisoning can be prevented by an intervention that both prevents a future increase in blood lead and reduces the risk of subclinical toxic effects for that particular child. This strategy therefore is protective against the future adverse outcome of poisoning or continued accumulation of subclinical effects ("secondary prevention") but comes too late to avoid the subclinical effects, which may already have been sustained.

Ideally, the preventive medicine model would screen houses, not children. Public health agencies have used elevated blood lead levels in children to identify housing with a lead paint problem. This approach is inappropriate. It is far better that houses be screened systematically for children's risk of lead exposure from living in unsafe homes; such screening would prevent clinical lead poisoning. Housing should be made safe for children; bad housing should not be identified by screening children. Children should not be used as markers to identify housing problems. Unfortunately, it is difficult to screen houses because of private property ownership rights and the right of access, the resources that would be required, and the very limited mandate of public health agencies when it comes to private homes.

The public health model is based on reducing risk for all members of a population, whether they are at high risk or not. Applied to lead, this approach is a lead toxicity prevention and elimination strategy. Concern for children today centers on reducing lead levels to as low as possible for all children. For background lead exposures, such as those described, the only practical intervention is to reduce exposure of all children in the population, treating the exposure as a risk factor. Children exposed in a multifactorial model may have a higher risk as a result of low levels of exposure, but their overall risk may be greater or less than that of other children, depending on their total risk profile. In the public health model, the benefit of investing limited funds in programs to reduce exposure to one risk factor must be compared with other potential investments (eg, reduction of exposure to mercury) on the basis of practicality, feasibility, and resources available.

Ideally, public health agencies should implement all three strategies. In practice, they cannot. Where should priorities be placed? Washington,

DC, provides an example. It is an old city with an unremediated housing stock. For such cities, it may be necessary in the short term to concentrate on preventing lead poisoning, a goal that, paradoxically, may not be achieved by lead elimination strategies alone. Mean blood lead levels continue to fall in Washington [31], as in the rest of the country [19], showing that lead intake from other sources is declining overall. The persistence of elevated blood lead levels and rare instances of symptomatic lead poisoning demonstrate that the major sources of lead have not yet been adequately controlled, however.

Lead elimination efforts have no obvious end, because in the modern environment there always will be sources of lead, released and deposited since the Industrial Revolution, and there is no threshold at which point remediation can be called entirely effective. Eventually, in public health agencies lead elimination efforts will come into budgetary and resource competition with efforts to reduce other risk factors for neurobehavioral outcomes and other public health priorities.

Acknowledgments

Melissa Greer assisted with editorial production.

References

[1] Flegal AR, Smith DR. Measurements of environmental lead contamination and human exposure. Rev Environ Contam Toxicol 1995;143:1–45.
[2] Tanner TH. Definition and mode of action of poisons. In: Toxicological memoranda. London: Henry Penshaw; 1878. p. 1.
[3] United States Department of Health and Human Services. Healthy people 2010. Washington, DC: US Government Printing Office; 2000.
[4] Stedman's on-line medical dictionary. Available at: http://www.stedmans.com/AtWork/section.cfm/45. Accessed March 30, 2007.
[5] Hodgson E. A textbook of modern toxicology. 3rd edition. Hoboken (NJ): John Wiley; 2004.
[6] Klaasen CD, Watkins JBI, editors. Casarett and Doull's essentials of toxicology. New York: McGraw-Hill/Medical Pub. Div; 2003.
[7] Timbrell JA. Introduction to toxicology. 3rd edition. New York: Taylor & Francis; 2002.
[8] National library of medicine. Toxnet-lead profile. Available at: Toxnet.nlm.nih.gov/cgi-bin/sis/search/f?/temp/~oxbxye:1:BASIC. Accessed May 15, 2004.
[9] National Institute of Environmental Health Sciences. NIEHS factsheet: what is lead poisoning? Available at: http://www.niehs.nih.gov/oc/factsheets/lyh/leadpoisn.htm. Accessed May 15, 2004.
[10] Centers for Disease Control and Prevention. Preventing lead poisoning in young children. Atlanta, GA. 2005. Available at: http://www.cdc.gov/nceh/lead/publications/PrevLeadPoisoning.pdf. Accessed February 10, 2007.
[11] Centers for Disease Control and Prevention. Blood lead levels surveillance 1997–2001. MMWR Surveill Summ 2003;52(SS10):1–21.
[12] Centers for Disease Control and Prevention. Lead poisoning associated with use of traditional ethnic remedies - California, 1991–1992. MMWR 1993;42(27):521–4.

[13] Agency for Toxic Substances and Disease Registry. Toxicological profile for lead. Atlanta (GA): ASTDR; 2004.

[14] American Academy of Pediatrics Committee on Drugs. Treatment guidelines for lead exposure in children. Pediatrics 1995;96:155–60.

[15] Environmental Protection Agency. FAQ-lead poisoning. Available at: www.epa.gov/region02/faq/lead_p.htm. Accessed May 15, 2004.

[16] Coalition to end childhood lead poisoning. Facts about lead poisoning. Available at: www.leadsafe.org/Parents/facts.html. Accessed May 15, 2004.

[17] National Safety Council. Understanding lead terminology. Available at: http://www.nsc.org/library/facts/lead.htm. Accessed March 30, 2007.

[18] Warren C. Brush with death: a social history of lead poisoning. Baltimore (MD): Johns Hopkins University Press; 2000. p. 178–225.

[19] Schwemberger JG, Mosby JE, Doa MJ, et al. Blood lead levels—United States, 1999–2002. MMWR Morb Mort Week Rep 2005;54(20):513–6.

[20] Bellinger DC. Lead. Pediatrics 2004;113:1016–22.

[21] Dietrich KN, Ris MD, Succop PA, et al. Early exposure to lead and juvenile delinquency. Neurotoxicol Teratol 2001;23:511–8.

[22] Lanphear BP, Dietrich KN, Auinger P, et al. Cognitive deficits associated with blood lead concentrations <10 microg/dL in US children and adolescents. Public Health Rep 2000; 115:521–9.

[23] Sawyer MG, Mudge J, Carty V, et al. A prospective study of childhood emotional and behavioural problems in Port Pirie, South Australia. Aust N Z J Psychiatry 1996;30:781–7.

[24] Tellez-Rojo MM, Bellinger DC, Arroyo-Quiroz C, et al. Longitudinal associations between blood lead concentrations lower than 10 microg/dL and neurobehavioral development in environmentally exposed children in Mexico City. Pediatrics 2006;118:e323–30.

[25] Lanphear BP, Hornung R, Khoury J, et al. Low-level environmental lead exposure and children's intellectual function: an international pooled analysis. Environ Health Perspect 2005; 113:894–9.

[26] Tong IS, Lu Y. Identification of confounders in the assessment of the relationship between lead exposure and child development. Ann Epidemiol 2001;11:38–45.

[27] Wigle DT. Child health and the environment. Oxford (UK): Oxford University Press; 2003.

[28] Rose G. The strategy of preventive medicine. Oxford (UK): Oxford University Press; 1992.

[29] Dietrich KN, Ware JH, Salganik M, et al. Effect of chelation therapy on the neuropsychological and behavioral development of lead-exposed children after school entry. Pediatrics 2004;114:19–26.

[30] Rogan WJ, Dietrich KN, Ware JH, et al. The effect of chelation therapy with succimer on neuropsychological development in children exposed to lead. N Engl J Med 2001;344: 1421–6.

[31] Stokes L, Onwuche NC, Thomas P, et al. Blood lead levels in residents of homes with elevated lead in tap water—District of Columbia, 2004. MMWR Morb Mort Week Rep 2004;53(12):268–70.

ELSEVIER
SAUNDERS

PEDIATRIC CLINICS
OF NORTH AMERICA

Pediatr Clin N Am
54 (2007) 237–269

Mercury Exposure and Public Health

Jack C. Clifton II, MD, MS

*Great Lakes Center for Children's Environmental Health, John H. Stroger,
Jr. Hospital of Cook County, Chicago, IL, USA*

Mercury is a metal that is a liquid at room temperature. The chemical symbol, Hg, is derived from "hydrargyros," the Greek for "water silver." Mercury may be found in one of three oxidation states, each with a specific toxic profile. In the zero oxidation state, Hg^0, elemental mercury exists as the liquid metallic form or as vapor. The two other inorganic forms of mercury are the mercurous (Hg^+) or the mercuric (Hg^{++}). The mercuric state may also form organic compounds such as methyl-, ethyl-, phenyl- or dimethylmercury.

Mercury has a long and interesting history deriving from its use in medicine and industry, with the resultant toxicity produced. In high enough doses, all forms of mercury can produce toxicity. Cinnabar (mercuric sulfide), the natural form of mercury, was used for the red coloring in cave drawings thousands of years ago. Tombs adorned with elemental mercury have been noted in Egypt dating back over 3500 years. Mercury's medicinal use probably originated in China and India nearly 2000 years ago. Since the Middle Ages, medications containing this element have been used as antibacterials (syphilis), antiseptics, dermatologic ointments, teething compounds, laxatives, and diuretics. In the United States in the 1800s, the etiology of an epidemic within the hat industry referred to as "hatters' shakes" or "Danbury shakes" resulted from mercury exposure that occurred during production of felt. The central nervous system (CNS)-based neurological and behavioral changes from this chronic exposure to mercury in poorly ventilated rooms were depicted in the Mad Hatter in Lewis Carroll's *Alice's Adventures in Wonderland*. Through the 1800s, children were commonly administered oral elemental mercury as a laxative. In the late 1800s and early to mid-1900s, infants who received calomel (Hg_2Cl_2) powders for the treatment of gum discomfort or ascariasis were noted to

---

All references preceded by a W refer to supplemental references available at: www.pediatric. theclinics.com.

E-mail address: jack_clifton@rush.edu

doi:10.1016/j.pcl.2007.02.005
pediatric.theclinics.com

develop acrodynia or pink disease. The most devastating tragedies related to mercury toxicity in recent history include Minamata Bay and Niagata, Japan in the 1950s and Iraq in the 1970s. More recent mercury toxicity issues include the extreme toxicity of the dimethylmercury compound noted in 1998, the possible toxicity related to dental amalgams, and the disproved relationship between vaccines and autism related to the presence of the mercury-containing preservative, thimerosal.

Elemental/metallic mercury

Sources

Exposure to Hg^0 may occur via inhalation, ingestion, and parenteral or subcutaneous administration. Hg^0 exists as both a liquid and vapor at room temperature. Exposure to the vapor may come from sources including the burning of fossil fuels, emissions from volcanic activity, smelting processes in mining activities, the industrial electrolytic production of HCl and NaOH, industrial and medical waste incineration, degassing from the natural erosion of the Earth's crust, evaporation from water, vaporization from dental amalgams, and crematoriums [1,2]. Exposure to elemental mercury in the liquid form may occur because of the mercury found in thermometers, barometers, disk batteries, dental amalgams, fluorescent light bulbs, sphygmomanometers, gas regulators, topical medications, cathartics, and substances used in magico-religious practices [3,W1,W2].

Pharmaco-toxicokinetics

Children are most commonly exposed to Hg^0 vapor via inhalation, accidental ingestion, and dental amalgams. The primary route of absorption of elemental mercury is via inhalation of the vapor, which readily transits across the pulmonary alveolar membranes, enters the circulation, and distributes to most tissues, including the red blood cells (RBCs), liver, and brain. This rapid diffusion from air to blood occurs because elemental mercury is an uncharged, lipid-soluble, intermediate-size atom. In the RBCs, the intracellular catalase oxidizes the Hg^0 to the divalent form, Hg^{++} [2,W3–W5], which complexes to protein, especially the hemoglobin, through reaction with the sulfhydryl groups. Even though the Hg^0 vapor remains in its elemental form in the body for only a few minutes, the catalase reaction is saturable, and the diffusion into the RBCs is not so rapid as to remove all of the solubilized mercury vapor instantly; therefore, a proportion of the vapor still dissolved in the blood is able to reach and cross the blood-brain barrier into the CNS [4–6]. In the CNS, catalase oxidizes Hg^0 to Hg^{++}, the presumed proximate agent of toxicity. This charged mercuric species is retained within the brain tissue, in some cases for many years. In the brain, numerous intracellular processes may be affected, including DNA,

RNA, and protein synthesis; microtubular polymerization; cell division; and cell migration [7,8,W6–W13]. Within several hours following inhalational exposure, all remaining Hg^0 is converted to Hg^{++}, and the toxic effects are also the same as those of Hg^{++}. (See the pharmaco-toxicokinetics section on inorganic mercury in this article.)

Whereas 97% of the absorption of the vapor occurs via the lungs, only 3% diffuses across the skin [9]. Volunteer studies using radioactive mercury vapor have estimated that 75% to 80% of the mercury inhaled is retained within the body [4,10]. In adult subjects following inhalation of mercury vapor, approximately 9 hours is required to reach a peak plasma concentration, with an estimated 4% of the retained dose present in the plasma at that time. The same study also found 4% to 10% of the Hg^0 was exhaled within 7 to 10 days following exposure [4,10]. Approximately 7% is distributed across the blood-brain barrier into the CNS, and 80% of the total body burden is deposited in the kidney as metallothionein-bound Hg^{++} [11,12,W8,W9].

The overall half-life in adults is approximately 60 days (range 36–100 days). The rapidity of the disappearance of mercury from the blood following vapor exposure is caused by the quick penetration of other body tissues. Therefore, Hg blood levels would be elevated only with a recent exposure. Excretion from the body takes place via the renal and fecal routes [13]. The urine mercury levels may not peak for days to a few weeks following the peak blood levels. In adults who have chronic occupational exposure, there may be a long time period of 6 to 10 months of accumulation in the kidney before the Hg excretion in the urine actually rises.

Elemental mercury inhaled by a pregnant woman also has the ability to cross the placenta, with subsequent concentration in the fetus as mercury bound to metallothionein [14,15,W5,W14–W16]. The fetus, especially in later gestation, seems to possess the same ability to oxidize elemental mercury to the divalent form via the catalase system, especially during first pass through the liver [W14,W15]. A study showed that inorganic Hg^{++}, originating as Hg^0 from maternal amalgam exposure with subsequent oxidation to Hg^{++}, accumulated in the placenta bound to metallothionein at a concentration four times that found in the maternal blood [16,W14]. Another study [W16], however, revealed that the mercury was most highly concentrated in the fetal liver and kidney as Hg^{++}, with much less in the brain; the catalase that is concentrated in the fetal liver may actually protect the fetal brain from Hg^0 by conversion to Hg^{++}, which cannot cross the fetal blood-brain barrier very well [W16]. Therefore, the fetal brain may not be at as high of a risk for toxicity from Hg^0 inhalation by the mother as compared with the fetal risk seen with methylmercury (MeHg) exposure in the mother; this conclusion seems to be supported by other studies [17,18].

Following ingestion, systemic absorption of elemental mercury in either liquid or vapor form is considered to be minimal ($<0.01\%$) in the individual with a normal gastrointestinal (GI) tract, with elimination occurring in the feces [19,20]; however, absorption may be increased in individuals with GI motility prolongation, as seen with accompanying anticholinergic poisoning, or with anatomic changes such as fistulae or perforations [21]. Absorption into the systemic circulation may also follow the subcutaneous deposition, intravenous administration, or aspiration of elemental mercury.

Toxicity

Hg^0 vapor exposure for a long enough time period at a high enough concentration will lead to organ damage in the brain, kidney, and lungs. Overall, inhalation of the vaporized elemental mercury is much more hazardous to human health than ingestion of the liquid form. If aspirated, either directly or as a result of vomiting, severe pulmonary compromise may follow, with resultant endobronchial damage and even death [22]. Intravenous (IV) administration, usually as an attempted suicide, may lead to pulmonary embolism with acute respiratory failure [14,23,24,W17–W26]. Subcutaneous injection of Hg^0 may lead to local abscess and granuloma formation associated with a prolonged systemic absorption, which necessitates local removal [25,26,W21,W22].

Exposure to elemental mercury vapor may occur in the residential, educational, industrial, or occupational setting, and may constitute an acute or chronic process [14,27,28,W20,W23–W31]. In one review of mercury exposures [29], 37% of these spills occurred in schools and private residences. Fourteen percent of the total mercury exposures occurred in the elementary and secondary schools, where nearly one half were caused by children playing with the mercury. Nearly 75% of the private residence exposures were caused by a spilled container of mercury or children playing with the metallic substance [29].

Homes can be contaminated when thermometers, manometers, and natural gas regulators are broken in the home, and when mercury is brought into the home and sprinkled or burned for religious or magical purposes. Mercury can be brought into the home on clothing or shoes, when children play with the mercury or when adults are exposed via poorly managed workplace mercury spills, such as when a sphygmomanometer breaks in a medical office [30].

Children in developing countries have also been exposed to mercury (Hg^0) vapor from local gold mining operations or from the burning of gold amalgam [31,32,W32–W34].

In the residential setting, children are at much greater exposure risk because elemental mercury vapor tends to settle to the floor, which is in much closer proximity to the breathing zone of the toddler or infant crawling on the floor. Acute exposure to Hg^0 vapor in the home may come from a spill, as previously cited, with the subsequent attempted cleanup using a vacuum cleaner. This agitation increases the aerosolization of the Hg^0, and the heat increases the vaporization of the elemental metal; the result is an increased exposure to the inhabitants of the home [33,34,W25,W29]. Acute exposure to vapor may produce some CNS effects caused by the small amount of unoxidized Hg^0 that may cross the blood-brain barrier. The more common symptoms that may occur within hours of inhalational exposure include a metal fume-fever type of presentation (metallic taste in the mouth, fever, chills, and dyspnea), nausea, vomiting, diarrhea, and cough along with chest tightness [35]. With exposure to high concentrations of elemental mercury vapor, toxicity to the renal system, including acute tubular necrosis (ATN) and acute renal failure (ARF), or to the pulmonary system, including an acute necrotizing bronchitis with subsequent progression to complete respiratory compromise and death, may occur [33,34,36,W29]. High level Hg^0 vapor inhalation with subsequent pulmonary embarrassment is the major cause of pediatric mortality with regard to elemental exposures [37,38,W35–W38].

Chronic exposure to mercury vapor primarily results in neurological effects in the CNS, which may not develop for weeks to months after exposure initiation [39]. Symptoms may include insomnia, intention tremor, stomatitis, gingivitis, loosened teeth, delusions, hallucinations, and mercurial erethism characterized by loss of memory, excitability, emotional lability, and extreme shyness. In addition, headache, visual changes (tunnel vision), peripheral neuropathy, and ataxia may result [40,41]. Autonomic dysfunction may manifest as excessive sweating and salivation. With chronic Hg^0 exposure, as in the occupational setting, Hg^{++} deposition in the kidney may lead to renal toxicity manifested as proteinuria (albumin, retinol binding protein) or nephrotic syndrome. In addition to the above symptoms, acrodynia may also be seen in children [42–44,W39,W40].

Inorganic mercury

Sources

Inorganic mercury compounds containing the Hg_2Cl_2 (mercurous) or $HgCl_2$ (mercuric) salts have been used as skin lightening creams (6%–10% Hg_2Cl_2), antiseptics, antibacterials, diuretics, teething discomfort "calomel" powders (Hg_2Cl_2, sweet mercury), and cathartics [45,46,W39]. Nonmedicinal applications of these salts include the use as detonators in explosives (mercuric fulminate, $Hg[OCN_2]$) and as paint pigments (HgS or vermilion). Even though many of these preparations, including the teething powders and skin lightening creams, are no longer available in the United States, these compounds are still present in other countries.

Pharmaco-toxicokinetics

Subsequent to ingestion, mercuric (Hg^{++}) and mercurous (Hg^+) inorganic salts are primarily absorbed in the duodenum of the GI tract [47]. Being more water-soluble and dissociable than calomel (mercurous salt), the mercuric chloride ($HgCl_2$) salt is more fully absorbed in the GI tract. The total absorption probably only approaches 10% to 15% in adults, but may be greater in the infant [48]; however, this absorption may be increased with mucosal damage secondary to the very caustic nature of the mercuric salt. The actual mechanism of absorption of Hg^{++} is still not known, but for years has been postulated to depend on the intestinal content [49]. The presence of thiol-containing compounds, such as glutathione (GSH) or amino acids derived from the diet, provides ligands in the GI lumen to which the Hg^{++} binds. These Hg-S-ligand complexes, because of their molecular "mimicry" of particular amino acids or peptides, are postulated to then be absorbed by active or passive mechanisms via the numerous amino acid and peptide transporters known to be located in the wall of the intestine [50–52,W41–W45]. The portal vein carries the Hg^{++} to the liver, where the Hg-conjugate probably transverses the sinusoidal membrane via one of the many amino acid transporters into the hepatocyte [53,54,W46,W47].

The kidney is the site of highest concentration of the mercuric Hg^{++} cation, where 90% of the total body load at steady state may be bound in the renal cortex by the Hg^{++}-inducible metallothionein (MT). The presence of this metal within the tubular cell may be seen within a few hours postingestion [55].

In most cases, after systemic absorption there is very little placental uptake and accumulation of Hg^{++}; but Hg^{++} may be found to enter this site [16,56]. In light of the fact that amino acid transporters are present in the placenta, molecular mimicry of an amino acid by the Hg^{++}-thiol conjugate may also allow for the accumulation of the metal within the placenta [57,58,W48].

Penetration of the blood-brain barrier by the ionic Hg^{++} is minimal ($< 0.01\%$). It is also felt that with a prolonged chronic exposure accompanied by a slow enough elimination, a small percentage of the inorganic mercuric form may actually be reduced back to the elemental form; thereby allowing passage into the brain, with accumulation in the cortices of the cerebellum and cerebrum.

The half-life of inorganic mercury appears to be approximately 40 days, with a range of 30 to 60 days. Excretion occurs primarily in the urine and feces. Normally, only about 10% of inorganic mercury excretion occurs via the kidney [59]; however, as Hg^{++} accumulates in the kidney with higher and prolonged exposures, renal excretion increases [60,61]. The GI tract is also critical to the elimination of Hg^{++}. Following a single oral dose of Hg^{++}, excretion is primarily by the fecal route. Two mechanisms for fecal elimination of the metal, both of which probably using transporter systems, include the bile transport of Hg^{++} into the intestinal lumen, and the enterocytic secretion of Hg^{++} derived from the blood into the intestinal lumen [53,62–65,W49–W53].

Toxicity

Acute ingestion of mercuric salts, whether accidentally or intentionally, must be considered potentially fatal, especially with a concentration of the salt in excess of 10% to 20%. Almost immediately following ingestion, the mucous membranes may display a grayish discoloration caused by the precipitation of the proteins within the membranes, associated with a metallic taste and pain in the oropharyngeal region. In addition, the patient usually experiences nausea, vomiting, and diarrhea, which may be accompanied by abdominal pain as a result of GI ulceration or possibly perforation. Hematemesis and hematochezia may be prominent, leading to massive fluid loss with complete circulatory collapse and death. Because of the caustic nature of the mercuric salts, the intestinal mucosa may be greatly compromised, allowing extensive systemic absorption of mercury, with subsequent concentration in the kidneys and a resultant acute tubular necrosis and renal failure.

Chronic poisoning is rare outside of occupational exposure to Hg^0 vapor, with subsequent conversion to Hg^{++} within the body; however, chronic exposure from products such as skin lightening cream, soaps, and teething discomfort powders may produce signs and symptoms similar to those noted with other forms of mercury intoxication, including generalized fatigue, weight loss, peripheral paresthesias, nephrotoxicity, cutaneous hyperpigmentation, and psychiatric abnormalities [66,67,W54–W58]. The effects on the fetus and newborn from prenatal exposure of the mother using these type of products are unstudied; however, the fetus may be at risk [68]. Pink disease or acrodynia, as well as erethism, have also been reported in infants or children following chronic exposure to the inorganic mercury contained within calomel teething powders (mercurous, Hg_2Cl_2), phenylmercuric acetate fungicides used by diaper services to rinse diapers, and phenylmercuric acetate fungicides in latex paints [69–71,W59–W62]. Chronic exposure may also lead to membranous glomerulonephritis or nephrotic syndrome through the immune-based production of auto-antibodies recognizing the glomerular basement membrane [72,73,W54,W63,W64]. An interstitial granulomatous nephritis has also been reported [74].

Organic mercury

Sources

The most common organic mercury compounds to which children and adults are exposed include methyl mercury, ethyl mercury, and phenyl mercury. All three have found uses as some form of biocide or antiseptic (Merthiolate [Eli Lilly, Indianapolis, Indiana] and Mercurochrome, no longer available in the United States). Methyl mercury (MeHg), the most familiar because the presence of this compound in fish and other seafood, represents the major source of organic mercury exposure for all individuals [75,76,W65–W68]. Because of the biomagnification of MeHg up the food chain, the highest concentrations of MeHg are found in the large, long-lived predatory fish, including pike, walleye, bass, tuna, tilefish, swordfish, shark, jack mackerel, and in whales [77,78,W31,W69–W73]. Upon ingestion, these

MeHg-contaminated fish then become the major organic mercury exposure for humans [79]. MeHg was at the center of the Minamata Bay poisoning through contaminated fish ingestion, and the Iraqi poisoning caused by the use of this compound as a fungicide on seed grain that accidentally found its way into the food supply. From these two catastrophes it was apparent that following ingestion of high doses of MeHg, toxicity to the brain, kidney, and immune system resulted [80–82]. It also became apparent that the developing brain of the fetus was much more sensitive to the neurotoxic effects of MeHg than the adult brain.

Other exposure sources of organic mercury include ethylmercurithiosalicylate, phenylmercuric acetate, phenylmercuric nitrate, and dimethyl mercury. Ethylmercurithiosalicylate has been used in the past as a topical antiseptic (Merthiolate) and as the preservative (thimerosol) in many vaccines. Phenylmercuric acetate and phenylmercuric nitrate found use in the paint industry for their anti-mildew properties, resulting in color preservation of the paint after surface application. Because of cases of toxicity, these mercury-containing compounds are no longer used in these products; newly manufactured indoor latex paint sold commercially has not contained any mercury since 1990 [W59]. Dimethyl mercury, used as a solvent in certain research laboratories, constitutes rare mercury exposures; however, this compound displays great toxicity [83].

Pharmaco-toxicokinetics

Subsequent to the ingestion of food contaminated with MeHg, the major route of human exposure, approximately 95% of the MeHg (CH_3Hg^+) released is absorbed in the GI tract [84–86,W31]. The CH_3Hg^+ is most likely absorbed from the GI lumen as a MeHg-cysteine (CH_3Hg-S-Cys) or MeHg-cysteine-glycine (CH_3Hg-S-CysGly) conjugate [87–89,W51,W74–W78], and absorption is very rapid [85]. More than 90% of MeHg found in the blood is concentrated in the RBCs in a ratio of 10–20:1 versus the concentration in the plasma [85,90,91,W42,W79–W84]. Following absorption from the duodenum, the CH_3Hg^+ travels to the liver, where the MeHg may then be taken up [92]. Distribution of MeHg to all the tissues within the body is very rapid, with steady state reached within 2 to 3 hours [19,93]. The primary targets of CH_3Hg^+ with resultant adverse clinical manifestations include the CNS and the placenta [94,W31]. From animal studies, it has been postulated that the thiol conjugate, CH_3Hg-S-Cys, structurally mimics methionine, which then allows this conjugate to cross the blood-brain barrier [93,95–97,W83–W93]. The mercury level within the brain may be three to six times the levels in the blood [98]. Once within the brain, MeHg appears to be very slowly biotransformed to Hg^{++}; whether the proximate toxin is Hg^{++} or MeHg is debated, but most likely is the CH_3Hg^+ [99,100,W94–W100]. The other important target tissue site of CH_3Hg^+ is the placenta. CH_3Hg^+ is known to cross the placental barrier and concentrate in both the placenta and the developing fetus, resulting in deleterious neurotoxicological outcomes [16,53,56,101–106,W89–W91,W101–W109].

The kidney may also be damaged by CH_3Hg^+ [99,107–110,W110–W113]. The renal proximal tubular cells may take up the MeHg in a way similar to the renal handling of Hg^{++} involving GSH [77,111–113,W114–W124].

Excretion of approximately 1% of the total body burden of MeHg per day occurs via both the fecal route and the renal route, with urinary excretion constituting less than 10% of the total body elimination [64,89,114–116,W49–W51,W125–W138]. The mean half-life in blood is 40 to 50 days, whereas whole body elimination is 70 to 80 days [1,85,86,104,117,118,W138,W139]. The GI excretion of MeHg in the feces by the breast-fed infant may be limited, however, in light of animal data reporting that demethylating bacteria may not become established in the lumen of the GI tract until after weaning, resulting in the reabsorption by the breast-fed infant's enterocytes of most of the MeHg secreted in the bile [92,119–121,W126,W140,W141].

The pharmaco-toxicokinetic characteristics of ethylmercury (EtHg) have not been as extensively evaluated as those of MeHg. EtHg is much more rapidly cleared from the blood, with a half-life of 7 to 10 days; therefore, the accumulation of EtHg within the body would not be expected when exposures are intermittent and separated by a time period greater than 1 to 2 months, as seen with immunization administration [122,123]. EtHg is metabolized much more quickly to divalent Hg^{++} than MeHg [19]. Murine models reveal that the distribution within the body is similar between MeHg and EtHg, but following equivalent doses of each in the same murine models, EtHg resulted in higher levels of total mercury in the kidney and blood and lower CNS mercury levels than those produced by MeHg. Brain damage was less and kidney damage was greater following EtHg exposure [107,124,125]. EtHg probably does not possess the ability to cross the blood-brain barrier via a process involving a transporter as seen with MeHg, but rather is dependent upon simple diffusion to enter the brain [93]. In rat studies, MeHg tends to produce more widely diffuse damage in the CNS, whereas EtHg was found to induce more patchy damage in the granular cell layer of the cerebellum [107]. Therefore, in comparison with MeHg, EtHg's reduced ability to cross the blood-brain barrier and produce CNS toxicity relates to its larger size, more rapid body clearance, lower bond energy between the carbon atom and Hg, allowing a more rapid production of the charged Hg^{++}, and reliance upon simple diffusion, rather than an active transport, for entrance into the brain [19,93,107,122,126–128,W142]. In addition, because of the more rapid clearance of EtHg from the blood, accumulation in the body would not occur as readily as noted with MeHg [122–124].

Toxicity

Organic mercury toxicity is related to the particular compound, its dose, the exposure route, and the age of the person at the time of the exposure.

Consumption of contaminated fish is the major exposure route for organic mercury in humans. MeHg poisoning is usually referred to as Minamata disease. MeHg's ability to cross both the blood-brain barrier and the placenta allow for serious toxicity in the person exposed, and in the case of the pregnant female, the fetus. The developing brain appears to suffer the most extensive damage from exposure to MeHg, a known teratogen [129–131]. Because of MeHg's formation of mercaptide bonds through the sulfhydryl groups of proteins, such as tubulin among others, neuronal cell migration and division within the CNS are adversely affected [130–134,W143]. At high-level MeHg exposure, neuronal and glial cell loss occur throughout the cortices of both the cerebrum and cerebellum, leading to devastating neurological defects in the infant [1,84,90,93,131,135–137,W144–W157]. The peripheral nervous system may also demonstrate damage, with the spinal posterior sensory roots being more affected than the anterior roots [131,138,139,W149]. Numerous biochemical processes have been postulated to be involved in MeHg neurotoxicity [140–142,W13,W31,W133,W152, W158–W161].

The toxicity of MeHg may be examined as acute or chronic high-dose exposures as well as chronic low-dose exposures. The chronic high-dose exposure of humans is well-illustrated in the 1953 to 1956 epidemic near Minamata Bay, Kumamoto Prefecture, Japan, and along the Agano River, Niigata Prefecture, Japan in 1964 to 1965, secondary to the ingestion of fish contaminated with MeHg [103,143,144]. The severity of the neurological sequelae from these exposures to MeHg became very apparent, especially when the exposure occurred prenatally from the mother ingesting the contaminated fish. Completely asymptomatic or only mildly toxic mothers gave birth to infants exhibiting or subsequently developing severe neurological dysfunction, demonstrating the difference between the adult and fetus in susceptibility of the CNS to MeHg exposure, with subsequent production of Minamata disease [145,146]. The resultant manifestations of fetal or congenital Minamata disease in these children included mental retardation, primitive reflexes, hyperkinesis, deafness, blindness, cerebral palsy, cerebellar ataxia, seizures, strabismus, dysarthria, and limb deformities [103–105, 144,147–149,W101,W146–W148]. Different pathological findings among exposed adults, children, and fetuses were revealed during autopsy evaluation with regard to cortical atrophy, corpus callosum hypoplasia, pyramidal tract demyelination, and hypoplasia of the cerebellar granular cell layer [90,103,150–152,W109,W162–W164]. The incidence of this congenital condition in the region of Minamata Bay between 1955 and 1958 was estimated to be nearly 30% of infants born to mothers who had been exposed [105].

A second mass poisoning with MeHg occurred in the early 1970s in rural Iraq, where MeHg fungicide-treated seed specified for planting was instead ground into flour, which was subsequently baked into bread that was consumed by the local population. This incident involved a more acute and higher-dose MeHg exposure than that seen in Minamata Bay. The children who were exposed prenatally displayed very similar CNS pathological changes and physical findings as those in Minamata Bay, including blindness, deafness, cerebral palsy, and paralysis [131,145]. Subsequent follow-up of the children who were exposed in utero revealed severe neurodevelopmental delays [104,145].

High-dose exposures such as those at Minamata Bay and in Iraq are rare [W100]. The major concern today is the possible neurotoxic effects of chronic low-level MeHg exposure, including those children exposed in utero from mothers who consume large amounts of contaminated fish during pregnancy.

A number of epidemiological investigations, including three longitudinal and several cross-sectional studies, have looked at a variety of neurological, neurodevelopmental, neuropsychiatric, and neurophysiologic end points in children prenatally exposed to mercury who were born to mothers exposed to chronic low doses of dietary MeHg [153–155,W165–W171]. One longitudinal study and two of the cross-sectional investigations found a significant relationship between prenatal MeHg exposure and any developmental outcome; the other nine studies, including two longitudinal investigations, revealed the absence of any significant relationship. A recent excellent review of most of these studies has been published [156].

The prospective epidemiologic studies which are referenced most frequently with regard to chronic, low-dose MeHg-associated neurotoxicity include the Seychelles Islands Study, with the pilot commenced in 1987 and the main study in 1989 [157–159,W71,W172–W183], and the Faroe Islands study initiated in 1986 [160–163,W168,W169,W184–W198]. These studies attempted to evaluate the possible association between the occurrence of adverse neurodevelopmental outcomes in children and chronic, low-dose MeHg exposure in utero secondary to maternal ingestion of fish contaminated with MeHg.

At the 7-year follow-up evaluation, the Faroe Islands study results revealed no significant association between MeHg exposure and neurophysiologic abnormalities or the functional neurological examination; however, there did appear to be a significant association of prenatal MeHg exposure (cord-blood MeHg) and deficits in the attention, language, and memory tests, even after controlling for the confounder polychlorinated biphenyl (PCB) content of the ingested whale blubber. At 14 years of follow-up, evaluation of the neurophysiologic data at that time as well as reanalysis of the 7-year neurophysiologic data revealed a significant association between the abnormalities in the brain stem auditory evoked potential (BAER) latencies and maternal hair Hg levels; confirming a lasting neurotoxic effect after intrauterine MeHg exposure [W166]. The Seychelles Study, however, through 9 years of follow-up in the evaluation of chronic, low-dose MeHg exposure to the fetus, was unable to define any statistically significant adverse neurodevelopmental outcomes in the children.

The explanation for the different outcomes of these two longitudinal studies in which the children appear to be exposed to similar levels of MeHg is unknown; however, possible explanations offered include genetic differences between the two populations, different MeHg sources, different types of exposure, and the presence of PCBs in the Faroe Islands diet, because some investigators report finding a synergism between PCBs and MeHg in the neurodevelopmental outcomes of MeHg-exposed children [W101,W168].

Regarding the toxicity of EtHg in humans, local hypersensitivity type reactions caused by the EtHg content in vaccines have been seen [164,165]. More severe toxicity, including acrodynia, renal failure, and neuropathies, have been noted subsequent to accidental poisonings, with high-level exposures to EtHg contained in such products as intravenously administered hepatitis B immunoglobulin and gamma globulin, dermally applied antiseptics for neonatal omphalocele treatment, orally ingested disinfectants, and aurally instilled medication for ear infection treatment [69,166–168,W199,W200]. In addition, toxicity similar to that of MeHg was noted to follow the ingestion of rice, bread, or pork contaminated with EtHg [W201–W203].

Management of mercury toxicity

A complete history and physical examination, including a detailed environmental and parental occupational history, are required for any suspected Hg intoxication. Confirmation of the exposure and the acute or chronic nature of the exposure should be ascertained. Identification of the source of Hg and removal from exposure is crucial. The subacute presentation of mercury toxicity may be very challenging. Any patient who has an altered mental status and renal failure requires a workup for mercury intoxication. As always, the ABCs need to be followed. The airway, breathing, and cardiovascular status of the patient must be assessed and stabilized as necessary. Decontamination must include removal of clothes as necessary, with washing of the skin with soap and water in the case of dermal exposure. Copious flushing of the eyes with normal saline should be performed if there has been an ocular exposure.

In the case of Hg^0 inhalation or aspiration, respiratory compromise with resultant failure may quickly ensue. Therefore, the patient's respiratory status must be monitored closely, including oxygen saturation. If the patient is symptomatic, a CXR and ABG are indicated, and preparation for intubation and subsequent conventional or high-frequency ventilation should be made. If the patient requires intubation, subsequent endotracheal suction for removal of any liquid Hg^0 in the airway is indicated as a decontamination procedure to reduce total exposure. In the event of IV injection of Hg^0, again the respiratory status as above needs to be of primary concern because of the possibility of pulmonary emboli. In the case of subcutaneous injection of Hg^0, if well-localized in the skin, surgical excision may be indicated to stop any further possible absorption. Ingestion of Hg^0 in the absence of vomiting or aspiration is usually fairly benign in the patient with a normal GI tract, and can usually be managed conservatively with observation for passage out of the body. KUBs may be used to monitor movement through the GI tract. Whole bowel irrigation (WBI) may be considered in these patients as well, but no good studies in this setting have been performed examining this modality.

In the case of inorganic Hg ingestion, such as $HgCl_2$, the patient must be approached as any other serious caustic ingestion, because of the severe mucosal damage with subsequent perforation that may occur after such an exposure. With acute GI toxicity, ABCs and supportive care are critical. In the symptomatic patient, aggressive fluid management after placement of large-bore IVs should be initiated in anticipation of the possible loss of large volumes of fluid with circulatory collapse. ENT should be consulted to evaluate the airway for burns, erosions, or caustic-induced injury that will allow the physician to anticipate early intubation, which may need to be surgically executed. Surgical consultation is also important in the management of an acute abdomen from perforation, which may occur anywhere along the GI tract. GI consultation for burn staging via endoscopy should also be requested. The symptomatic patient should be kept NPO and should not be lavaged or receive any activated charcoal until both the laryngopharyngeal region and the GI tract have been evaluated. Once the GI tract and vocal cords have been deemed uninjured, activated charcoal may be considered in light of the in vitro evidence that $HgCl_2$ actually does bind to charcoal in a ratio of 800 mg $HgCl_2$ to 1 g of activated charcoal [169]. In the small child, even with an intact GI tract, orogastric lavage should not be performed because of the size of tube required. Lavage with protein-containing solutions (milk or egg whites) to help complex mercury has been experimented with, but not adequately studied.

The target organs for inorganic Hg toxicity include not only the GI tract, but because of its accumulation in the proximal tubular cells, the kidneys. Renal function must be scrutinized for oliguric or anuric renal failure that would require hemodialysis.

Laboratory evaluation specifically focusing on the confirmation of mercury exposure may include the 24-hour urine, whole blood or RBC Hg levels, and hair Hg levels. Urine levels are also critical for the appropriate monitoring of effective chelation therapy in the Hg-intoxicated patient. The urine collection for Hg should be done in a metal-free, acid-washed polyethylene container with no preservatives. Normal 24-hour urine mercury levels should be below 20 mcg/L. Above this level, evidence for excessive Hg exposure exists. With urine levels greater than 100 to 150 mcg/L, subtle neurological signs may be found; levels greater than 300 mcg/L are usually associated with overt symptoms. All blood for Hg determination should be collected in a metal-free EDTA tube. Whole blood mercury levels are usually less than 10 to 20 mcg/L.

Because MeHg is concentrated in the RBC and eliminated mostly through secretion into the GI tract and feces in the bile, the 24-hour urine level is not very useful; however, the whole blood level is a good measure of the body burden for MeHg and should be collected. Whole blood mercury levels may be as high as 200 mcg/L in the patient who consumes large amounts of fish, especially those varieties known to contain elevated MeHg levels. In the case of inorganic mercury, specifically Hg^{++}, because of its accumulation in the kidney and excretion in the urine, the 24-hour urine level is the gold standard for inorganic mercury exposure. In that Hg^0 is oxidized rapidly to Hg^{++} with excretion in the urine, the 24-hour urine level should also be collected, especially in chronic exposures. Because EtHg, the metabolic product of thimerosal, may be rapidly metabolized to Hg^{++}, a 24-hour urine collection is indicated. Mercury blood levels after Hg^0 inhalation or inorganic Hg exposure may be helpful only if collected soon after the exposure, because inorganic mercury is rapidly distributed to the tissues with return of levels to normal within 1 or 2 days. Hair levels may be a very reliable measure for MeHg exposure because MeHg is most highly concentrated at that site, with a hair:blood ratio of approximately 250:1 [170]; however, these hair levels of mercury may represent past exposures as well as external environmental contamination. Along with the possible inconsistencies in hair Hg measurements among various laboratories, this measure should never be used alone, but always in conjunction with the whole blood level for MeHg [171,172].

Once exposure of the patient to Hg has been determined as discussed above, the major goal, in addition to removing the patient from the source, is to remove the Hg from the patient in an attempt to prevent or reduce toxicity. Enhancement of elimination of Hg using hemodialysis (HD) or peritoneal dialysis (PD) most likely has no role in the treatment of mercury toxicity in terms of removing the mercury from the body, because mercury binds to proteins, and in the case of MeHg, enters the CNS. Therefore, removal by these two techniques is very inefficient [173]; however, HD may play a major role in inorganic Hg toxicity in the treatment of the ensuing renal failure.

In the symptomatic Hg-intoxicated patient, immediate chelation therapy is indicated. Because Hg may concentrate in the blood, CNS, and kidneys, an attempt to chelate the metal and increase its excretion constitutes a rational plan;. however, whether this course of treatment actually benefits the severely intoxicated patient is not completely known. In addition, the indications for chelation are not completely established, except for the patient who has the clinical presentation consistent with severe Hg toxicity or the laboratory evidence of a large total mercury body load [174].

All of the chelators that have been used in the treatment of Hg toxicity possess sulfhydryl groups; hence, they become competitors of blood and tissue proteins for the binding of Hg. Overall, the chelators will increase Hg excretion in the urine, but their effectiveness in decreasing toxicity in the patient is not as certain. Urine levels may then be monitored to follow the effectiveness and the course of chelator treatment. If chelation is being considered, a clinical toxicologist should always be consulted for appropriate dosing and side effect monitoring.

Chelation in the acute inorganic Hg (Hg^0 or Hg^{++})-poisoned patient may be accomplished with dimercaprol (BAL), D-penicillamine (DPCN), dimercaptopropane sulfonate (DMPS), or succimer (DMSA). There is currently no Food and Drug administration (FDA)-approved chelator for MeHg or EtHg toxicity. Chelation should be reserved for severe intoxication. Both BAL and DPCN have been shown to be effective in MeHg toxicity in rat studies when administered within 24 hours of the MeHg injection [175]; however, BAL is absolutely contraindicated in the treatment of organic mercury toxicity, because some animal studies revealed an increased mobilization of Hg into the brain [176]. N-acetylcysteine (NAC) administered orally as a chelator for MeHg and inorganic mercury poisoning has been studied only in animals [115,177]. DMPS was noted to have reduced the blood half-life of MeHg in poisoned patients in Iraq in 1971; however, clinical improvement was not observed [115,178]. DMSA is presently the most frequently used chelator in the treatment of severe MeHg poisoning. DMSA is superior to DPCN in increasing urinary excretion of Hg in chronic MeHg poisoning. DMSA was also found to be superior to DMPS in decreasing brain Hg and increasing urinary Hg in a MeHg-poisoned murine model [179]. In addition to the oral administration, DMSA's minimal side-effect profile also makes it the best option for MeHg poisoning treatment.

Special considerations

Mercury and autism

In addition to the debate regarding the relationship between low- level MeHg exposure and neurodevelopment, further debate implicating mercury as a neurotoxicant in children arose with the hypothesis that the occurrence of autistic spectrum disorders was caused by the presence in vaccines of the mercury-containing preservative, thimerosal. Thimerosal, 49.6% mercury by weight as the sodium salt of ethylmercurithiosalicylate, was the preservative used in a variety of pharmaceuticals and multidose vials of vaccines since the 1930s [180–182,W204,W205]. Thimerosal is metabolized to EtHg and thiosalicylate with the subsequent rapid production of Hg^{++} [19]. Most children in the. United States who received four diptheria-pertussis-tetanus (DPT) doses, four Hemophilus influenza type b (Hib) doses and three hepatitis B (Hep B) doses would have been administered a total EtHg dose of approximately 187.5 mcg to 237.5 mcg in the first 6 months to 2 years of life [183–185]. In light of the apparently increased incidence of autism in the 1990s, along with the increased mercury exposure through the childhood vaccination program in the United States, the hypothesis of thimerosal-containing vaccines as an etiology for autism seemed plausible to some, but anecdotal to others [186–188,W204,W205,W206–W218]. In July, 1999, the U.S. Public Health Service, the U.S. Department of Health and Human Services, and the American Academy of Pediatrics (AAP) stated that the amount of mercury that accumulated in the child during administration of the infant vaccines exceeded the 1997 U.S. Environmental Protection Agency (EPA) guidelines [2,189,190]; however, no toxic effects had ever been noted except for a delayed type hypersensitivity reaction [164,165]. They called for a reduction or elimination of the mercury-containing preservative from vaccines and for the immediate discontinuation of the hepatitis B vaccine administered to children born to low-risk mothers until an acceptable alternative thimerosal-free vaccine became available. The 1997 EPA guidelines pertained specifically to cumulative oral exposures of MeHg, not parenterally administered EtHg. Because of the paucity of data in 1999 regarding the pharmacokinetics and toxicity of EtHg and thimerosal, these recommendations were based on the assumption of similar pharmacotoxicologic characteristics for EtHg and MeHg, as well as the exposure to EtHg in childhood vaccines being cumulative in nature. This assumption is incorrect, however, as previously discussed in the section on the pharmaco-toxicokinetics of EtHg. In 2001, after reviewing all pertinent data, including a retrospective cohort study investigating several years of pediatric data from several health maintenance organizations (HMOs) in the United States, the Institute of Medicine's (IOM) Immunization Safety Review Committee stated "the evidence is inadequate to accept or reject a causal relationship between exposure to thimerosal from vaccines and the neurodevelopmental disorders of autism, ADHD [attention deficit hyperactivity disorder], and speech or language delay." Even though the evidence was inadequate, the hypothesis was deemed "biologically plausible" by this Committee [184,191,W218]. Therefore, more research, including a better understanding of the pharmacokinetics of EtHg, was called for by the Committee. Subsequently, several epidemiologic studies attempted to further evaluate the possible relationship between mercury-containing vaccines and autism [192–195,W207,W219–W223]. A few of these studies supported a relationship; however, methodological flaws and biases precluded the validity of this claim [192,193,W221,W222]. The majority of the studies did not provide epidemiologic evidence for an association between thimerosal-containing vaccines and autism. A recent excellent review of these studies has been published [196].

Neurotoxic effects of high-dose EtHg and thimerosal are postulated to be similar to high-dose MeHg, as demonstrated by the clinical symptoms reported in several diverse exposures, including those noted in patients subsequent to the ingestion of bread made from seeds treated with EtHg p-toluene sulfonanilide in Iraq, those following the ingestion of pork from a pig fed seeds treated with EtHg, and those subsequent to the consumption of tainted rice in China [148,166–168,197,198,W199,W203]. In vitro systems using high-dose thimerosal exposure have revealed its ability to increase oxidative stress, deplete GHS stores similar to MeHg, and induce apoptosis. Neuronal cells have also been found to be more sensitive than astrocytes [199,200,W224,W225]. The effects of low-dose EtHg, however, are not completely known.

In 2004, the Immunization Safety Review Committee of the IOM reconsidered the possible relationship between autism and thimerosal-containing vaccines. Based on the more recently published epidemiological data, the IOM shifted from the position of neutrality to the conclusion that "the evidence favors rejection of a causal relationship between thimerosal-containing vaccines and autism" [201]. Since the 2004 report, two cohort studies from the United Kingdom examining the relationship between thimerosal contained within vaccines and the occurrence of neurodevelopmental disorders have been published; the conclusions reached from both of these studies are in agreement with the 2004 IOM statement of no causal relationship [195,W219]. Since thimerosal-free DTaP vaccine approval in the U.S. in March, 2001, routinely recommended vaccines for children 6 years of age or under are free of thimerosal or contain only trace amounts of the EtHg component. Today, a 6-month-old infant is exposed to less than 3 mcg of mercury from a standard immunization schedule in the Unites States or the European Union (EU). Influenza vaccine without thimerosal is also available; however, influenza vaccines administered to pregnant women after the first trimester and Rho(D) immunoglobulin still contain thimerosal, as do the many vaccines administered to the pediatric population in developing countries. Actually, most countries continue to use vaccines with thimerosal as the preservative for children. The World Health Organization (WHO) endorses the use of thimerosal-containing vaccines for children on the basis that there are no convincing pharmacokinetic or epidemiological studies that have proven thimerosal-containing, vaccine-associated EtHg toxicity [202–204]. In addition, the economics of using thimerosal-free vaccines in developing countries may be prohibitive. Therefore, WHO feels that thimerosal-containing vaccine administration is much better than no vaccinations at all in these countries [205].

Because of the thimerosal-autism debate, some parents have chosen not to immunize their children out of the fear of mercury toxicity [206,207]. It is incumbent upon the pediatrician to relay accurate information regarding the absence of any studies defining any relationship between vaccinations and autism. The risk associated with not immunizing a child against preventable diseases greatly outweighs the unfounded risk associated with mercury toxicity from the vaccine. Because thimerosal-free vaccines are available in the United States there is no risk.

Dental amalgams

Dental amalgam for filling decayed posterior teeth has been in use since its introduction in the United States in 1830 [208,209]. The amalgam is an alloy composed of approximately 50% elemental mercury, along with other metals such as copper, silver, tin, zinc, or palladium. With its introduction into dentistry, there were immediate questions regarding the possible toxicity and health effects that the mercury-containing amalgam might have on the individual. In 1845, during the "first amalgam war," the American Society of Dental Surgeons requested from its members an oath to never use the amalgam. The "second amalgam war" was initiated in the 1920s by German chemists who once more questioned the safety of the amalgam because of the presence of mercury. In the late 1970s the "third amalgam war" began after the discovery that mercury concentrations within the oral cavity as a result of the release of Hg^0 vapor could approach air levels above the guidelines set for occupational exposure [209]. It became apparent, however, that the total amount of Hg that could possibly be inhaled and subsequently absorbed via the lungs was not large, because of the small volume of the oral cavity. The amount of Hg released has been estimated to be approximately 1.7 mcg/12 amalgams/day [210,211]; however, the Hg^0 released from the amalgams is absorbed and distributed within the body [212–214,W102,W226–W234]. Studies also discovered that mercury release from amalgams may increase during the activities of chewing, brushing the teeth, or nocturnal bruxism; individuals chewing excessively, as may be seen with the use of nicotine gum, may have urinary Hg levels approaching the occupational health limits [210,215–217,W235–W239]. Examination of urinary mercury concentrations in individuals who had amalgams and who were not excessive gum chewers were found to be quite small compared with individuals who were occupationally exposed to Hg vapor, but greater than those who did not possess amalgams. Occupationally exposed individuals may have urinary Hg concentrations of 20 to 50 mcg/L, whereas non-occupationally exposed individuals who have amalgams may typically have Hg concentrations of 2 to 4 mcg/L [218–221,W236,W240–W245]. It has been estimated that the urine Hg level will rise by approximately 1 mcg/L for every 10 amalgam surfaces an individual possesses [W241]. Because amalgams constitute the major non-occupational source of exposure to Hg^0, with a resultant very small increase in urinary Hg levels, the question arises as to the possible toxicity of chronic low-level exposure to mercury vapor. Several epidemiological studies have investigated any possible link between this type of mercury exposure and human disease, including amyotrophic lateral sclerosis (ALS), multiple sclerosis (MS), Parkinson's disease, and Alzheimer's disease. The available scientific evidence reveals no link between amalgams and clinical toxicity [222–224,W246,W247]. Another retrospective study also revealed the absence of any association between the presence of amalgam fillings and cognitive dysfunction [225]. The National Institutes of Health (NIH) has also stated that there is no personal health risk imposed by the presence of amalgams, and that replacement with a non-amalgam polymer to reduce mercury exposure is not indicated [226]. Until recently, prospective randomized clinical trials examining the relationship between amalgam mercury exposure and adverse clinical effects had not been published. One randomized controlled trial over a 7-year period of time attempted to assess any differences in the health effects in 507 children, ages 8 to 10 years old, who received posterior dental restorations using either a mercury-based dental amalgam or resin composite-based material [227,228]. Even though there was a significantly higher level of mercury in the urine of those children receiving the mercury-based amalgam restorations, no significant difference was found between the two groups in neurobehavioral assessments (memory; attention/concentration; motor/visuomotor) or nerve conduction velocity studies. A second randomized clinical trial, the New England Children's Amalgam Trial (NECAT), compared the health effects in children receiving mercury-based amalgam posterior dental restorations with those in children receiving resin composite material. Five hundred thirty-four children, ages 6 to 10 years old, were followed over 5 years using the full-scale IQ test on the Wechsler Intelligence Scale for Children-Third Edition (WISC-III) for neuropsychological evaluation and measuring urine albumin for renal function evaluation. Even though a significantly higher mercury level after 5 years was found in the urine of the amalgam group of children, no significant difference between the two groups was noted in terms of neuropsychological measurements (full-scale IQ; memory or visuomotor scores) or urinary albumin levels [229,230]. Even though these two pediatric studies reveal no significant health effects associated with the placement of mercury-based amalgam, one cannot conclude that there is no risk, because of some of the limitations of these studies [231]. In an attempt to study any amalgam-related mercury toxicity in children (6–10 years old at enrollment), the 5-year Children's Amalgam Trial is presently assessing the change in IQ scores over the 5 years, along with neuropsychological parameters and renal function, in the children receiving amalgam in comparison with those receiving mercury-free composite materials for their posterior restorations [230]. Overall, even though dental amalgam is a source of low-level exposure to mercury, at this time there is no scientifically-based evidence indicting amalgam as the etiology for clinical toxicity, except for the rare local hypersensitivity reaction [232,233].

Breast milk, nutritionally beneficial to the neonate, may also be a deposit for contaminants within the environment [234,235]. The question regarding the detrimental effects to the breast-fed infant by mercury transferred into the milk from the Hg^0 vapor originating from maternal amalgams has been considered. On one hand, investigators felt that the breast-fed infant was at risk [212,236,237,W227], whereas other researchers felt that the presence of amalgams posed no risk to the fetus or infant [238–240]. Most studies, with the exception of two [241,242], agree that the total amount of Hg within breast milk is significantly correlated with the amalgam number of the mother [212,236,238,239,243]. One study, looking at a low fish-consuming population of women, found a significant correlation between breast milk Hg concentration and the maternal amalgam surface number. After measurement of the Hg concentration within the breast milk of these women and assuming a 21-day old, 4 kg infant with a breast milk intake of approximately 150 g milk/kg/day, these investigators estimated the Hg intake by the infants would exceed the adult WHO reference values for Hg intake (0.5 mcg/kg/day) in 56.5% of the cases, thereby exposing the infant to an excess amount of mercury [243,244]. Another study in low fish-consuming women found that total and inorganic Hg in both the blood and breast milk also correlated with the number of amalgams possessed by the mother. Using similar calculations as above, based on body mass, the highest Hg intake in these infants was 0.3 mcg/kg/day [212]; however, the true exposure of the breast -fed baby must depend upon the amount of mercury that is actually absorbed through the infant's GI tract into the systemic circulation. Knowing that MeHg is very well-absorbed by the GI tract, whereas inorganic mercury is not, the species of mercury present in the milk would most likely in part affect the level of actual "exposure" that the infant experiences subsequent to the ingestion of the breast milk. Although Hg^{++} absorption via the adult GI tract is thought to be low, Hg^{++} may have a greater uptake by the infant GI tract [48,245]. Breast milk-to-plasma ratios for inorganic Hg of 0.6-1, along with the finding that breast milk mercury levels appear to be correlated with the maternal blood inorganic mercury concentration, would seem to demonstrate the transport of inorganic mercury into the breast milk [120,212,246]. Even though the mercury levels in the milk may be elevated, if the majority of this Hg is present as the inorganic type (Hg^{++}) derived from the amalgam exposure, the actual amount of Hg that enters the infant's system may be negligible, with minimal risk of toxicity. One study reported the mean percentage of inorganic mercury in breast milk to be 55%, with a range of 16% to 100% [212]. Other factors that may affect Hg levels in breast milk that need to be considered include the age of the mother and the timing of the study in relationship to the stage of lactation [239,247]. The proteins within breast milk that bind mercury are reported to be casein and albumin, with differential binding by inorganic or organic mercury [248]. During lactation, the total protein concentration within the breast milk actually declines between the colostrum and the later milk; total Hg content of breast milk has been noted to decrease during this same time period [234,248,249]. One study has also reported that the mercury content within colostrum is significantly correlated with the number of maternal amalgams; however, later in lactation the significance is no longer present [239]. So perhaps the risk of mercury toxicity to the infant, even if present early on in breast feeding, may not pose a risk as the child ages and the milk matures. The infant's capacity to secrete and excrete MeHg may also play a role. An animal model revealed the presence of bacteria within the GI lumen possessing the ability to enzymatically demethylate MeHg to Hg^{++} with a subsequent reduction in absorption of the MeHg. These bacteria, however, are not established in the rat GI tract until after weaning [W126,W140,W141]. If demethylation of MeHg within the GI tract of the human infant does not occur until after weaning, as seen in the animal model, then most of the MeHg in the breast milk, even if present in very low concentration, may be completely absorbed, leading to blood levels greater than expected in the baby. More research regarding neonatal GI Hg^{++} absorption and the species of mercury present in breast milk is obviously needed to properly answer the questions surrounding the risk of exposure to amalgam-derived mercury in breast-fed infants.

Fish consumption

Following the discovery of the high MeHg content of some fish, public concern and debate regarding possible mercury toxicity from fish ingestion arose. A large amount of research has focused on attempting to estimate how much mercury is actually ingested when consuming fish in the diet. This is a difficult area of investigation, because MeHg content may vary greatly within the same or between different species of fish, and the location where the fish reside when caught may also greatly influence the amount of MeHg within that particular type of fish. Questions addressed include how much MeHg should an individual be able to consume per day or per week, which fish and what amount of each type of fish may be safely eaten, and what are the guidelines for fish consumption in children, pregnant women, women who are of child-bearing age who may become pregnant, and women who are breastfeeding.

According to the FDA, the mercury content of fish in the United States ranges from 0.04 to 1.5 mcg/g fish (0.04–1.5 ppm), much below the levels found in fish from other countries [250]. The FDA set the safe exposure limit of MeHg in fish at 1 mcg/g fish (1 ppm), which is an order of magnitude lower than the lowest level associated with adverse effects [251]. Fish sold commercially in the United States must have a Hg content at or below this level; however, fish caught for sport may very well not meet these FDA requirements. In 1995, the FDA issued a top 10 list of safe seafood that could be consumed without any need for concern; these 10 composed approximately 80% of the market. The 10 fish, along with their mercury content in ppm, include: light canned tuna (0.206), shrimp (0.047), pollack (0.15), salmon (0.035), cod (0.121), non-farm–raised catfish (0.088), clams (0.023), flounder (0.092), crab (0.117), and scallops (0.042). The fish with much higher mercury content include shark, swordfish, king mackerel, and tilefish.

In light of the possible adverse health effects of mercury, a reference dose (RfD) of 0.1 mcg/kg body weight/day was set by the EPA. The RfD estimates the amount of mercury that an individual, including children in this case, may safely consume on a daily basis for an entire lifetime without fear of harmful effects. This RfD was actually derived by the National Research Council after considering many of the MeHg-related studies previously discussed in this article [252].

In counseling patients regarding fish intake so as to avoid possible mercury toxicity, physicians should follow the guidelines proposed by the EPA and FDA. The latest fish advisory issued jointly by the EPA and FDA in 2004 is specifically for "women who are pregnant, women who might become pregnant, nursing mothers, and young children" [253]. The advisory states that this group of individuals should not consume the fatty fish, including shark, swordfish, king mackerel, and tilefish. These individuals may consume up to 6 ounces/week (1 average meal) of albacore "white" tuna , which contains more mercury than canned light tuna, and locally caught fish from local lakes, rivers, and coastal areas. If locally caught fish is chosen, then the individual is not to eat any other fish that week. The advisory also states that these individuals may instead eat up to 12 ounces/week (two average meals) of a variety of fish and shellfish low in mercury, which includes any of those fish previously stated to be in the top 10 fish list above. Most recently, the Institute of Medicine of The National Academies also investigated the benefits and risks associated with seafood. The Committee on Nutrient Relationships in Seafood concurred with the EPA and FDA recommendations for fish consumption [254].

References

[1] Clarkson TW. Mercury: major issues in environmental health. Environ Health Perspect 1993;100:31–8.
[2] US Environmental Protection Agency. Mercury study report to congress, volume IV: an assessment of exposure to mercury in the United States; 1997.
[3] Gibson R, Taylor TS. Nicor says mercury spilled at more sites. Contamination found at 6 new locations, company tells state. Chicago Tribune (Chicago Sports Final Edition); 2000.
[4] Hursh JB, Greenwood MR, Clarkson TW, et al. The effect of ethanol on the fate of mercury vapor inhaled by man. Pharmacol Exp Ther 1980;214(3):520–7.
[5] Jonsson F, Sandborgh-Englund G, Johanson G. A compartmental model for the kinetics of mercury vapor in humans. Toxicol Appl Pharmacol 1999;155(2):161–8.
[6] Clarkson TW, Halbach S, Magos L, et al. On the mechanism of oxidation of inhaled mercury vapor. In: Bhatnagar R, editor. Molecular basis of environmental toxicity. Ann Arbor (MI): Science Pub; 1980. p. 419–27.
[7] Leong CC, Syed NI, Lorscheider FL. Retrograde degeneration of neurite membrane structural integrity of nerve growth cones following in vitro exposure to mercury. Neuroreport 2001;12(4):733–7.
[8] Panda D, Miller HP, Wilson L. Rapid treadmilling of brain microtubules free of microtubule-associated proteins in vitro and its suppression by tau. Proc Natl Acad Sci U S A 1999; 96(22):12459–64.
[9] Hursh JB, Clarkson TW, Miles EF, et al. Percutaneous absorption of mercury vapor by man. Arch Environ Health 1989;44(2):120–7.
[10] Hursh JB, Cherian MG, Clarkson TW, et al. Clearance of mercury (HG-197, HG-203) vapor inhaled by human subjects. Arch Environ Health 1976;31(6):302–9.
[11] Berlin M. Dose-response relation and diagnostic indices of mercury concentrations in critical organs upon exposure to mercury and mercurials. In: Nordberg G, editor. Effects and dose-response relationships of toxic metals. Amsterdam: Elsevier Science Publisher; 1979. p. 387–445.

[12] Roels HA, Boeckx M, Ceulemans E, et al. Urinary excretion of mercury after occupational exposure to mercury vapour and influence of the chelating agent meso-2,3-dimercaptosuccinic acid (DMSA). Br J Ind Med 1991;48(4):247–53.

[13] Sandborgh-Englund G, Elinder CG, Johanson G, et al. The absorption, blood levels, and excretion of mercury after a single dose of mercury vapor in humans. Toxicol Appl Pharmacol 1998;150(1):146–53.

[14] Ask K, Akesson A, Berglund M, et al. Inorganic mercury and methylmercury in placentas of Swedish women. Environ Health Perspect 2002;110(5):523–6.

[15] Newland MC, Warfvinge K, Berlin M. Behavioral consequences of in utero exposure to mercury vapor: alterations in lever-press durations and learning in squirrel monkeys. Toxicol Appl Pharmacol 1996;139(2):374–86.

[16] Dencker L, Danielsson B, Khayat A, et al. Deposition of metals in embryo and fetus. In: Clarkson T, editor. Reproductive and developmental toxicity of metals. New York: Plenum Press; 1983. p. 607–37.

[17] Clarkson TW. The pharmacology of mercury compounds. Annu Rev Pharmacol 1972;12: 375–406.

[18] Bornmann G, Henke G, Alfes H, et al. [Intestinal absorption of metallic mercury]. Archiv fur Toxikologie 1970;26(3):203–9 [in German].

[19] Bredfeldt JE, Moeller DD. Systemic mercury intoxication following rupture of a Miller-Abbott tube. Am J Gastroenterol 1978;69(4):478–80.

[20] Zimmerman JE. Fatality following metallic mercury aspiration during removal of a long intestinal tube. JAMA 1969;208(11):2158–60.

[21] Eyer F, Felgenhauer N, Pfab R, et al. Neither DMPS nor DMSA is effective in quantitative elimination of elemental mercury after intentional IV injection. Clin Toxicol (Phila) 2006; 44(4):395–7.

[22] Gutierrez F, Leon L. Images in clinical medicine. Elemental mercury embolism to the lung. N Engl J Med 2000;342(24):1791.

[23] Smith SR, Jaffe DM, Skinner MA. Case report of metallic mercury injury. Pediatr Emerg Care 1997;13(2):114–6.

[24] Cole JK, Holbrook JL. Focal mercury toxicity: a case report [see comment]. J Hand Surg [Am] 1994;19(4):602–3.

[25] George L, Scott F. The Mercury emergency in Hamilton, September 1993. J Environ Health 1996;58(8):4–6.

[26] Fagala GE, Wigg CL. Psychiatric manifestations of mercury poisoning. J Am Acad Child Adolesc Psychiatry 1992;31(2):306–11.

[27] Zeitz P, Orr MF, Kaye WE. Public health consequences of mercury spills: Hazardous Substances Emergency Events Surveillance system, 1993–1998. Environ Health Perspect 2002; 110(2):129–32.

[28] Baughman TA. Elemental mercury spills. Environ Health Perspect 2006;114(2):147–52.

[29] Snodgrass W, Sullivan JB Jr, Rumack BH, et al. Mercury poisoning from home gold ore processing. Use of penicillamine and dimercaprol. JAMA 1981;246(17):1929–31.

[30] Counter SA, Buchanan LH, Laurell G, et al. Blood mercury and auditory neuro-sensory responses in children and adults in the Nambija gold mining area of Ecuador. Neurotoxicology 1998;19(2):185–96.

[31] Moromisato DY, Anas NG, Goodman G. Mercury inhalation poisoning and acute lung injury in a child. Use of high-frequency oscillatory ventilation. Chest 1994;105(2):613–5.

[32] Rowens B, Guerrero-Betancourt D, Gottlieb CA, et al. Respiratory failure and death following acute inhalation of mercury vapor. A clinical and histologic perspective. Chest 1991; 99(1):185–90.

[33] Fuortes LJ, Weismann DN, Graeff ML, et al. Immune thrombocytopenia and elemental mercury poisoning. J Toxicol Clin Toxicol 1995;33(5):449–55.

[34] Aguado S, de Quiros IF, Marin R, et al. Acute mercury vapour intoxication: report of six cases. Nephrol Dial Transplant 1989;4(2):133–6.

[35] Moutinho ME, Tompkins AL, Rowland TW, et al. Acute mercury vapor poisoning. Fatality in an infant. Am J Dis Child 1981;135(1):42–4.

[36] Campbell JS. Acute mercurial poisoning by inhalation of metallic vapour in an infant. Can J Med 1948;58:72–5.

[37] Cherry D, Lowry L, Velez L, et al. Elemental mercury poisoning in a family of seven [erratum appears in Fam Community Health 2002 Apr;25(1):x]. Fam Community Health 2002;24(4):1–8.

[38] Buckell M, Hunter D, Milton R, et al. Chronic mercury poisoning. 1946. Br J Ind Med 1993;50(2):97–106.

[39] Neal PA, Jones RR. Chronic mercurialism in the hatter's fur cutting industry. JAMA 1938; 110:337.

[40] Satoh H. Occupational and environmental toxicology of mercury and its compounds. Ind Health 2000;38(2):153–64.

[41] Risher J, DeWoskin R. Agency for Toxic Substances and Disease Registry (ATSDR), 1999. Atlanta (GA): U.S. Dept Public Health; 1999. p. 824–33.

[42] Centers for Disease Control and Prevention (CDC), 1991. Current trends in acute and chronic poisoning from residential exposures to elemental mercury—Michigan, 1989–1990. MMWR Morb Mort Wkly Rep. 40:393–395.

[43] Boyd AS, Seger D, Vannucci S, et al. Mercury exposure and cutaneous disease. J Am Acad Dermatol 2000;43(1 Pt 1):81–90.

[44] DeBont B, Lauwerys R, Govaerts H, et al. Yellow mercuric oxide ointment and mercury intoxication. Eur J Pediatr 1986;145:217–8.

[45] Clarkson T. The uptake and disposition of inhaled mercury vapor. In: Potential biological consequences of mercury released from dental amalgam. Proceedings from a Conference. Stockholm; 1992.

[46] Foulkes EC. Transport of toxic heavy metals across cell membranes. Proc Soc Exp Biol Med 2000;223(3):234–40.

[47] Dave MH, Schulz N, Zecevic M, et al. Expression of heteromeric amino acid transporters along the murine intestine. J Physiol 2004;558(Pt 2):597–610.

[48] Laporte JM, Andres S, Mason RP. Effect of ligands and other metals on the uptake of mercury and methylmercury across the gills and the intestine of the blue crab (Callinectes sapidus). Comp Biochem Physiol C Toxicol Pharmacol 2002;131(2):185–96.

[49] Andres S, Laporte JM, Mason RP. Mercury accumulation and flux across the gills and the intestine of the blue crab (Callinectes sapidus). Aquat Toxicol 2002;56(4):303–20.

[50] Leslie EM, Deeley RG, Cole SP. Toxicological relevance of the multidrug resistance protein 1, MRP1 (ABCC1) and related transporters. Toxicology 2001;167(1):3–23.

[51] Keppler D, Leier I, Jedlitschky G, et al. ATP-dependent transport of glutathione S-conjugates by the multidrug resistance protein MRP1 and its apical isoform MRP2. Chemico-Biological Interactions 1998;111–112:153–61.

[52] Zalups RK. Early aspects of the intrarenal distribution of mercury after the intravenous administration of mercuric chloride. Toxicology 1993;79(3):215–28.

[53] Suzuki T, Matsumoto N, Miyama T, et al. Placental transfer of mercuric chloride, phenyl mercury acetate and methylmercury acetate in mice. Ind Health 1967;5:149–55.

[54] Jansson T. Amino acid transporters in the human placenta. Pediatr Res 2001;49(2): 141–7.

[55] Kudo Y, Boyd CA. Human placental amino acid transporter genes: expression and function. Reproduction 2002;124(5):593–600.

[56] Dales L, Kahn E, Wei E. Methylmercury poisoning. An assessment of the sportfish hazard in California. Calif Med 1971;114(3):13–5.

[57] Tan M, Parkin JE. Route of decomposition of thiomersal (thimerosal). Int J Pharm 2000; 208(1–2):23–34.

[58] Zalups RK, Lash LH. Advances in understanding the renal transport and toxicity of mercury. J Toxicol Environ Health 1994;42(1):1–44.

[59] Zalups RK. Intestinal handling of mercury in the rat: implications of intestinal secretion of inorganic mercury following biliary ligation or cannulation. J Toxicol Environ Health A 1998;53(8):615–36.

[60] Lien DC, Todoruk DN, Rajani HR, et al. Accidental inhalation of mercury vapour: respiratory and toxicologic consequences. Can Med Assoc J 1983;129(6):591–5.

[61] Campbell D, Gonzales M, Sullivan JB Jr. Mercury. In: Sullivan JBJ, Krieger GR, editors. Hazardous materials toxicology–clinical principles of environmental health. Baltimore (MD): Williams & Wilkens; 1992. p. 824–33.

[62] Clarkson TW. The three modern faces of mercury. Environ Health Perspect 2002; 110(Suppl 1):11–23.

[63] Ballatori N, Clarkson TW. Biliary transport of glutathione and methylmercury. Am J Physiol 1983;244(4):G435–41.

[64] Ballatori N, Clarkson TW. Dependence of biliary secretion of inorganic mercury on the biliary transport of glutathione. Biochem Pharmacol 1984;33(7):1093–8.

[65] Dyall-Smith DJ, Scurry JP. Mercury pigmentation and high mercury levels from the use of a cosmetic cream. Med J Aust 1990;153(7):409–10.

[66] Weldon MM, Smolinski MS, Maroufi A, et al. Mercury poisoning associated with a Mexican beauty cream. West J Med 2000;173(1):15–8 [discussion: 19].

[67] Lauwerys R, Bonnier C, Evrard P, et al. Prenatal and early postnatal intoxication by inorganic mercury resulting from the maternal use of mercury containing soap. Hum Toxicol 1987;6(3):253–6.

[68] Matheson DS, Clarkson TW, Gelfand EW. Mercury toxicity (acrodynia) induced by long-term injection of gammaglobulin. J Pediatr 1980;97(1):153–5.

[69] Dinehart SM, Dillard R, Raimer SS, et al. Cutaneous manifestations of acrodynia (pink disease). Arch Dermatol 1988;124(1):107–9.

[70] Astalfi A, Goelli C. Paper presented at the Monitereo Biologico: proceedings of Academia Nacional de Medicino de Buenos Aires Conference. Buenos Aires (Argentina), November 3, 1981.

[71] Soo YO, Chow KM, Lam CW, et al. A whitened face woman with nephrotic syndrome. Am J Kid Dis 2003;41(1):250–3.

[72] McRill C, Boyer LV, Flood TJ, et al. Mercury toxicity due to use of a cosmetic cream. J Occup Environ Med 2000;42(1):4–7.

[73] Franco A, Antolin A, Trigueros M, et al. Two consecutive episodes of acute renal failure following mercury poisoning. Nephrol Dial Transplant 1997;12(2):328–30.

[74] U.S. Department of Health and Human Services; 1994. Toxicological profile for mercury (update). TP-93/10. Washington, DC: U.S. DHHS.

[75] Bjerregaard P. Cardiovascular disease and environmental pollutants: the Arctic aspect. Arctic Med Res 1996;55(Suppl 1):25–31.

[76] Zalups RK. Molecular interactions with mercury in the kidney. Pharmacol Rev 2000;52(1): 113–43.

[77] Jensen S, Jernelov A. Biological methylation of mercury in aquatic organisms. Nature 1969; 223(207):753–4.

[78] Ratcliffe HE, Swanson GM, Fischer LJ. Human exposure to mercury: a critical assessment of the evidence of adverse health effects. J Toxicol Environ Health 1996;49(3): 221–70.

[79] Aschner M, Aschner JL. Mercury neurotoxicity: mechanisms of blood-brain barrier transport. Neurosci Biobehav Rev 1990;14(2):169–76.

[80] Kosuda LL, Hosseinzadeh H, Greiner DL, et al. Role of RT6+ T lymphocytes in mercury-induced renal autoimmunity: experimental manipulations of "susceptible" and "resistant" rats. J Toxicol Environ Health 1994;42(3):303–21.

[81] Loftenius A, Sandborgh-Englund G, Ekstrand J. Acute exposure to mercury from amalgam: no short-time effect on the peripheral blood lymphocytes in healthy individuals. J Toxicol Environ Health A 1998;54(7):547–60.

[82] Nierenberg DW, Nordgren RE, Chang MB, et al. Delayed cerebellar disease and death after accidental exposure to dimethylmercury [see comment]. N Engl J Med 1998; 338(23):1672–6.

[83] WHO. Methylmercury environmental health criteria 101. Geneva (France): International Programme on Chemical Safety, World Health Organization; 1990.

[84] Aberg B, Ekman L, Falk R, et al. Metabolism of methyl mercury (203Hg) compounds in man. Arch Environ Health 1969;19(4):478–84.

[85] Miettinen JK. Absorption and elimination of dietary (Hg++) and methylmercury in man. Mercury, mercurial and mercaptans. In: Miller MW, Clarkson TW, editors. Springfield (IL): C.C. Thomas; 1973. p. 233–46.

[86] Urano T, Iwasaki A, Himeno S, et al. Absorption of methylmercury compounds from rat intestine. Toxicol Lett 1990;50(2–3):159–64.

[87] Norseth T, Clarkson TW. Intestinal transport of 203Hg-labeled methyl mercury chloride. Role of biotransformation in rats. Arch Environ Health 1971;22(5):568–77.

[88] Wang W, Clarkson TW, Ballatori N. gamma-Glutamyl transpeptidase and l-cysteine regulate methylmercury uptake by HepG2 cells, a human hepatoma cell line. Toxicol Appl Pharmacol 2000;168(1):72–8.

[89] Clarkson TW. The toxicology of mercury. Crit Rev Clin Lab Sci 1997;34(4):369–403.

[90] Kershaw TG, Clarkson TW, Dhahir PH. The relationship between blood levels and dose of methylmercury in man. Arch Environ Health 1980;35(1):28–36.

[91] Thomas DJ, Smith JC. Effects of coadministered low-molecular-weight thiol compounds on short-term distribution of methyl mercury in the rat. Toxicol Appl Pharmacol 1982; 62(1):104–10.

[92] Kerper LE, Ballatori N, Clarkson TW. Methylmercury transport across the blood-brain barrier by an amino acid carrier. Am J Physiol 1992;262(5 Pt 2):R761–5.

[93] World Health Organization. Mercury. Air quality guidelines. 2nd edition. Copenhagen (Denmark): WHO Regional Office Europe; 2000. Chap. 69.

[94] Jernelov A. A new biochemical pathway for the methylation of mercury and some ecological implications. In: Miller MW, Clarkson TW, editors. Mercury, mercurials and mercaptans. Springfield (IL): Thomas; 1973. p. 315–24.

[95] Landner L. Biochemical model for the biological methylation of mercury suggested from methylation studies in vivo with Neurospora crassa. Nature 1971;230(5294): 452–4.

[96] Betz AL, Goldstein GW. Polarity of the blood-brain barrier: neutral amino acid transport into isolated brain capillaries. Science 1978;202(4364):225–7.

[97] Berlin M, Carlson J, Norseth T. Dose-dependence of methylmercury metabolism. A study of distribution: biotransformation and excretion in the squirrel monkey. Arch Environ Health 1975;30(6):307–13.

[98] Norseth T, Clarkson TW. Studies on the biotransformation of 203Hg-labeled methyl mercury chloride in rats. Arch Environ Health 1970;21(6):717–27.

[99] Syversen TL. Distribution of mercury in enzymatically characterized subcellular fractions from the developing rat brain after injections of methylmercuric chloride and diethylmercury. Biochem Pharmacol 1974;23(21):2999–3007.

[100] Inouye M, Kajiwara Y. Developmental disturbances of the fetal brain in guinea-pigs caused by methylmercury. Arch Toxicol 1988;62(1):15–21.

[101] Harada M. Minamata disease: methylmercury poisoning in Japan caused by environmental pollution. Crit Rev Toxicol 1995;25(1):1–24.

[102] Amin-Zaki L, Elhassani S, Majeed MA, et al. Intra-uterine methylmercury poisoning in Iraq. Pediatrics 1974;54(5):587–95.

[103] Harada M. Congenital Minamata disease: intrauterine methylmercury poisoning. Teratology 1978;18(2):285–8.

[104] Kajiwara Y, Inouye M. Effects of methylmercury and mercuric chloride on preimplantation mouse embryos in vivo. Teratology 1986;33(2):231–7.

[105] Magos L, Brown AW, Sparrow S, et al. The comparative toxicology of ethyl- and methyl-mercury. Arch Toxicol 1985;57(4):260–7.

[106] Friberg L. Studies on the metabolism of mercuric chloride and methyl mercury dicyandia-mide; experiments on rats given subcutaneous injections with radioactive mercury (Hg203). A M A Archives of Ind Health 1959;20(1):42–9.

[107] Inouye M, Murao K, Kajiwara Y. Behavioral and neuropathological effects of prenatal methylmercury exposure in mice. Neurobehav Toxicol Teratol 1985;7(3):227–32.

[108] Prickett CS, Laug EP, Kunze FM. Distribution of mercury in rats following oral and intra-venous administration of mercuric acetate and phenylmercuric acetate. Proc Soc Exp Biol Med 1950;73(4):585–8.

[109] Norseth T, Clarkson TW. Biotransformation of methylmercury salts in the rat studied by specific determination of inorganic mercury. Biochem Pharmacol 1970;19(10):2775–83.

[110] Richardson RJ, Murphy SD. Effect of glutathione depletion on tissue deposition of methylmercury in rats. Toxicol Appl Pharmacol 1975;31(3):505–19.

[111] Alexander J, Aaseth J. Organ distribution and cellular uptake of methyl mercury in the rat as influenced by the intra- and extracellular glutathione concentration. Biochem Pharmacol 1982;31(5):685–90.

[112] Tanaka T, Naganuma A, Miura N, et al. Role of testosterone in gamma-glutamyltranspep-tidase-dependent renal methylmercury uptake in mice. Toxicol Appl Pharmacol 1992;112(1):58–63.

[113] Clarkson TW, Friberg L, Nordberg G, et al. Biological monitoring of toxic metals. New York: Plenum Press; 1988.

[114] Koh AS, Simmons-Willis TA, Pritchard JB, et al. Identification of a mechanism by which the methylmercury antidotes N-acetylcysteine and dimercaptopropanesulfonate enhance urinary metal excretion: transport by the renal organic anion transporter-1. Mol Pharmacol 2002;62(4):921–6.

[115] Schaub TP, Kartenbeck J, Konig J, et al. Expression of the conjugate export pump encoded by the mrp2 gene in the apical membrane of kidney proximal tubules. J Am Soc Nephrol 1997;8(8):1213–21.

[116] Bernard S, Purdue P. Metabolic models for methyl and inorganic mercury. Health Phys 1984;46(3):695–9.

[117] Sherlock J, Hislop J, Newton D, et al. Elevation of mercury in human blood from con-trolled chronic ingestion of methylmercury in fish. Hum Toxicol 1984;3(2):117–31.

[118] Rowland I, Davies M, Grasso P. Biosynthesis of methylmercury compounds by the intes-tinal flora of the rat. Arch Environ Health 1977;32(1):24–8.

[119] Sundberg J, Jonsson S, Karlsson MO, et al. Kinetics of methylmercury and inorganic mer-cury in lactating and nonlactating mice. Toxicol Appl Pharmacol 1998;151(2):319–29.

[120] Grandjean P, Jorgensen PJ, Weihe P. Human milk as a source of methylmercury exposure in infants. Environ Health Perspect 1994;102(1):74–7.

[121] Clements CJ. The evidence for the safety of thiomersal in newborn and infant vaccines. Vaccine 2004;22(15–16):1854–61.

[122] Bigham M, Copes R. Thiomersal in vaccines: balancing the risk of adverse effects with the risk of vaccine-preventable disease. Drug Saf 2005;28(2):89–101.

[123] Magos L. Review on the toxicity of ethylmercury, including its presence as a preservative in biological and pharmaceutical products. J Appl Toxicol 2001;21(1):1–5.

[124] Suzuki T, Miyama T, Katsunuma H. Comparative study of bodily distribution of mercury in mice after subcutaneous administration of methyl, ethyl, and n-propyl mercury acetate. Jpn J Exp Med 1963;33:277–82.

[125] Magos L. Neurotoxic character of thimerosal and the allometric extrapolation of adult clearance half-time to infants. J Appl Toxicol 2003;23(4):263–9.

[126] Burbacher TM, Shen DD, Liberato N, et al. Comparison of blood and brain mercury levels in infant monkeys exposed to methylmercury or vaccines containing thimerosal. Environ Health Perspect 2005;113(8):1015–21.

[127] Pichichero ME, Cernichiari E, Loprelato J, et al. Mercury concentrations and metabolism in infants receiving vaccines containing thimerosal: a descriptive study. Lancet 2002;360: 1737–41.

[128] Hanson JW. Human teratology. In: Rimoin DL, Connor JM, Pyreritz RE, editors. Principles and practice of medical genetics, vol. 1. 3rd edition. New York: Churchill Livingston; 1997. p. 697–724.

[129] Albers JW, Kallenbach LR, Fine LJ, et al. Neurological abnormalities associated with remote occupational elemental mercury exposure. Ann Neurol 1988;24(5):651–9.

[130] Choi BH, Lapham LW, Amin-Zaki L, et al. Abnormal neuronal migration, deranged cerebral cortical organization, and diffuse white matter astrocytosis of human fetal brain: a major effect of methylmercury poisoning in utero. J Neuropathol Exp Neurol 1978; 37(6):719–33.

[131] Miura K, Imura N. Mechanism of methylmercury cytotoxicity. Crit Rev Toxicol 1987; 18(3):161–88.

[132] Rodier PM, Aschner M, Sager PR. Mitotic arrest in the developing CNS after prenatal exposure to methylmercury. Neurobehav Toxicol Teratol 1984;6(5):379–85.

[133] Philbert MA, Billingsley ML, Reuhl KR. Mechanisms of injury in the central nervous system. Toxicol Pathol 2000;28(1):43–53.

[134] Eto K, Takizawa Y, Akagi H, et al. Differential diagnosis between organic and inorganic mercury poisoning in human cases—the pathologic point of view. Toxicol Pathol 1999; 27(6):664–71.

[135] Castoldi AF, Coccini T, Ceccatelli S, et al. Neurotoxicity and molecular effects of methylmercury. Brain Res Bull 2001;55(2):197–203.

[136] Brown DL, Reuhl KR, Bormann S, et al. Effects of methyl mercury on the microtubule system of mouse lymphocytes. Toxicol Appl Pharmacol 1988;94(1):66–75.

[137] Eto K, Takeuchi T. Pathological changes of human sural nerves in Minamato disease (methylmercury poisoning). Light and electron microscopic studies. Virchows Arch B Cell Pathol 1977;23(2):109–28.

[138] Takeuchi T, Eto K, Oyanag S, et al. Ultrastructural changes of human sural nerves in the neuropathy induced by intrauterine methylmercury poisoning (so-called fetal Minamata disease). Virchows Arch B Cell Pathol 1978;27(2):137–54.

[139] Atchison WD, Hare MF. Mechanisms of methylmercury-induced neurotoxicity. FASEB J 1994;8(9):622–9.

[140] Miura K, Clarkson TW. Reduced methylmercury accumulation in a methylmercury-resistant rat pheochromocytoma PC12 cell line. Toxicol Appl Pharmacol 1993;118(1):39–45.

[141] Sager PR, Aschner M, Rodier PM. Persistent, differential alterations in developing cerebellar cortex of male and female mice after methylmercury exposure. Brain Res 1984;314(1): 1–11.

[142] Tsubaki T. Outbreak of intoxication by organic compounds in Niigata Prefecture. Jpn J Med 1967;6:132–3.

[143] Tsubaki T, Irukayama K. Minamata disease: Methylmercury poisoning in Minamata and Niigata, Japan. New York: Elsevier; 1977.

[144] Bakir F, Rustam H, Tikriti S, et al. Clinical and epidemiological aspects of methylmercury poisoning. Postgrad Med J 1980;56(651):1–10.

[145] Takeuchi T. Pathology of Minamata disease. With special reference to its pathogenesis. Acta Pathol Jpn 1982;32(Suppl 1):73–99.

[146] Takeuchi T, Eto N, Eto K. Neuropathology of childhood cases of methylmercury poisoning (Minamata disease) with prolonged symptoms, with particular reference to the decortication syndrome. Neurotoxicology 1979;1:1–20.

[147] Bakir F, Damluji SF, Amin-Zaki L, et al. Methylmercury poisoning in Iraq. Science 1973; 181(96):230–41.

[148] Kondo K. Congenital Minamata disease: warnings from Japan's experience. J Child Neurol 2000;15(7):458–64.

[149] Takeuchi T, Matsumoto H, Koya G. A pathological study on the fetal Minamata disease diagnosed clinically as so-called infantile cerebral palsy. Adv Neurol Sci 1964;8:145–61.

[150] Eto K. Minamata disease. Neuropathology 2000;20(Suppl):S14–9.

[151] Syversen T. Effects of methymercury on in vivo isolated cerebral and cerebellar neurons. Neuropathol Appl Neurobiol 1977;3:225–36.

[152] Cordier S, Garel M, Mandereau L, et al. Neurodevelopmental investigations among methylmercury-exposed children in French Guiana. Environ Res 2002;89(1):1–11.

[153] Grandjean P, White RF, Nielsen A, et al. Methylmercury neurotoxicity in Amazonian children downstream from gold mining. Environ Health Perspect 1999;107(7):587–91.

[154] Marsh DO, Turner MD, Smith JC, et al. Fetal methylmercury study in a Peruvian fish-eating population. Neurotoxicology 1995;16(4):717–26.

[155] Spurgeon A. Prenatal methylmercury exposure and developmental outcomes: review of the evidence and discussion of future directions. Environ Health Perspect 2006;114(2):307–12.

[156] Axtell CD, Myers GJ, Davidson PW, et al. Semiparametric modeling of age at achieving developmental milestones after prenatal exposure to methylmercury in the Seychelles Child Development Study. Environ Health Perspect 1998;106(9):559–63.

[157] Axtell CD, Cox C, Myers GJ, et al. Association between methylmercury exposure from fish consumption and child development at five and a half years of age in the Seychelles Child Development Study: an evaluation of nonlinear relationships. Environ Res 2000;84(2): 71–80.

[158] Cox C, Breazna A, Davidson PW, et al. Prenatal and postnatal methylmercury exposure and neurodevelopmental outcomes [comment]. JAMA 1999;282(14):1333–4.

[159] Grandjean P, Weihe P, Jorgensen PJ, et al. Impact of maternal seafood diet on fetal exposure to mercury, selenium, and lead. Arch Environ Health 1992;47(3):185–95.

[160] Grandjean P, Weihe P, White RF. Milestone development in infants exposed to methylmercury from human milk. Neurotoxicology 1995;16(1):27–33.

[161] Grandjean P, White RF, Sullivan K, et al. Impact of contrast sensitivity performance on visually presented neurobehavioral tests in mercury-exposed children. Neurotoxicol Teratol 2001;23(2):141–6.

[162] Grandjean P, Weihe P, White RF, et al. Cognitive deficit in 7-year-old children with prenatal exposure to methylmercury. Neurotoxicol Teratol 1997;19(6):417–28.

[163] Cox NH, Forsyth A. Thiomersal allergy and vaccination reactions. Contact Derm 1988; 18(4):229–33.

[164] Goncalo M, Figueiredo A, Goncalo S. Hypersensitivity to thimerosal: the sensitizing moiety. Contact Derm 1996;34(3):201–3.

[165] Fagan DG, Pritchard JS, Clarkson TW, et al. Organ mercury levels in infants with omphaloceles treated with organic mercurial antiseptic. Arch Dis Child 1977;52:962–4.

[166] Pfab R, Muckter H, Roider G, et al. Clinical course of seven poisonings with thimerosal. Clin Toxicol 1996;34:453–60.

[167] Rohyans J, Walson PD, Wood GA, et al. Mercury toxicity following merthiolate ear irrigations. J Pediatr 1994;104:311–3.

[168] Andersen AH. Experimental studies on the pharmacology of activated charcoal; III. adsorption from gastrointestinal contents. Acta Pharmacol 1948;4:275–84.

[169] Katz SA, Katz RB. Use of hair analysis for evaluating mercury intoxication of the human body: a review. J Appl Toxicol 1992;12(2):79–84.

[170] Sauder P, Livardjani F, Jaeger A, et al. Acute mercury chloride intoxication. Effects of hemodialysis and plasma exchange on mercury kinetic. J Toxicol Clin Toxicol 1988; 26(3–4):189–97.

[171] Seidel S, Kreutzer R, Smith D, et al. Assessment of commercial laboratories performing hair mineral analysis [see comment]. JAMA 2001;285(1):67–72.

[172] Gill US, Schwartz HM, Bigras L. Results of multiyear international interlaboratory comparison program for mercury in human hair. Arch Environ Contam Toxicol 2002;43(4): 466–72.

[173] Blanusa M, Varnai VM, Piasek M, et al. Chelators as antidotes of metal toxicity: therapeutic and experimental aspects. Curr Med Chem 2005;12(23):2771–94.

[174] Zimmer LJ, Carter DE. The efficacy of 2,3-dimercaptopropanol and D-penicillamine on methyl mercury induced neurological signs and weight loss. Life Sci 1978;23(10):1025–34.

[175] Berlin M, Rylander R. Increased brain uptake of mercury induced by 2,3-dimercaptopropanol (BAL) in mice exposed to phenylmercuric acetate. J Pharmacol Exp Ther 1964;146: 236–40.

[176] Ballatori N, Lieberman MW, Wang W. N-acetylcysteine as an antidote in methylmercury poisoning. Environ Health Perspect 1998;106(5):267–71.

[177] Clarkson TW, Magos L, Cox C, et al. Tests of efficacy of antidotes for removal of methylmercury in human poisoning during the Iraq outbreak. J Pharmacol Exp Ther 1981;218(1): 74–83.

[178] Aaseth J, Frieheim EA. Treatment of methyl mercury poisoning in mice with 2,3-dimercaptosuccinic acid and other complexing thiols. Acta Pharmacol Toxicol 1978;42(4):248–52.

[179] Wilson GS. The hazards of immunization. New York: The Athlone Press; 1967. p. 75–84.

[180] Bernier RH, Frank JA, Nolan TF. Abscesses complicating DTP vaccination. Am J Dis Child 1981;135:826–8.

[181] Simon PA, Chen RT, Elliot JA, et al. Outbreak of pyogenic abscesses after diptheria and tetanus toxoids and pertussis vaccine. Pediatr Infect Dis J 1993;12:368–71.

[182] Ball LK, Ball R, Pratt RD. An assessment of thimerosal use in childhood vaccines [see comment]. Pediatrics 2001;107(5):1147–54.

[183] Institute of Medicine. Immunization safety review: thimerosal-containing vaccines and neurodevelopmental disorders. In: Stratton K, Gable A, McCormick MC, editors. Under review: Thimerosol-containing vaccines and neurodevelopmental disorders. Washington, DC: National Academy Press; 2001. p. 27–37.

[184] Clements CJ, Ball LK, Ball R, et al. Thiomersal in vaccines. Lancet 2000;355(9211): 1279–80.

[185] Bernard S, Enayati A, Redwood L, et al. Autism: a novel form of mercury poisoning. Med Hypotheses 2001;56:462–71.

[186] Bernard S, Enayati A, Roger H, et al. The role of mercury in the pathogenesis of autism. Mol Psychiatry 2002;7(Suppl 2):S42–3.

[187] Kidd PM. Autism, an extreme challenge to integrative medicine. Part: 1: the knowledge base. Altern Med Rev 2002;7(4):292–316.

[188] Thimerosal in vaccines: a joint statement of the American Academy of Pediatrics and the Public Health Service. MMWR Morb Mortal Wkly Rep 1999;48:563–5.

[189] American Academy of Pediatrics, Committee on Infectious Diseases and Committee on Environmental Health. Thimerosal in vaccines—an interim report to clinicians. Pediatrics 1999;104:570–4.

[190] DeStefano F, Vaccine Safety Datalink Research Group. The Vaccine Safety Datalink project. Pharmacoepidemiol Drug Saf 2001;10(5):403–6.

[191] Geier MR, Geier DA. Neurodevelopmental disorders after thimerosal-containing vaccines: a brief communication [see comment]. Exp Biol Med 2003;228(6):660–4.

[192] Geier DA, Geier MR. An assessment of the impact of thimerosal on childhood neurodevelopmental disorders. Pediatr Rehabil 2003;6(2):97–102.

[193] Verstraeten T, Davis RL, DeStefano F, et al. Safety of thimerosal-containing vaccines: a two-phased study of computerized health maintenance organization databases. Pediatrics 2003;112(5):1039–48.

[194] Andrews N, Miller E, Grant A, et al. Thimerosal exposure in infants and developmental disorders: a retrospective cohort study in the United kingdom does not support a causal association. Pediatrics 2004;114(3):584–91.

[195] Parker SK, Schwartz B, Todd J, et al. Thimerosal-containing vaccines and autistic spectrum disorder: a critical review of published original data. Pediatrics 2004;114(3): 793–804.

[196] Suzuki T, Takemoto TL, Kashiwazaki H, et al. Metabolic fate of ethyl mercury in man and animal. In: Miller MW, Clarkson TW, editors. Mercury, mercurials and mercaptans. Springfield (IL): Charles C. Thomas; 1973. p. 208–40.

[197] Damluji S. Mercurial poisoning with the fungicide Granosan M. J Fac Med Bagdad 1962;4: 83–103.

[198] James SJ, Slikker W 3rd, Melnyk S, et al. Thimerosal neurotoxicity is associated with glutathione depletion: protection with glutathione precursors. Neurotoxicology 2005;26(1): 1–8.

[199] Baskin DS, Ngo H, Didenko VV. Thimerosal induces DNA breaks, caspase-3 activation, membrane damage, and cell death in cultured human neurons and fibroblasts. Toxicol Sci 2003;74(2):361–8.

[200] Institute of Medicine. Immunization safety review: vaccines and autism. Washington, DC: National Academy Press; 2004.

[201] World Health Organization. Global Advisory Committee on Vaccine Safety, 2003 Jun 11–12. Wkly Epidemiol Rec 2003;32:282–4.

[202] World Health Organization. WHO Guidelines on regulatory expectations related to the elimination, reduction or replacement of thimerosal in vaccines: technical report series (unnumbered); 2003.

[203] World Health Organization. Global Advisory Committee on Vaccine Safety: statement on thimerosal; 2003.

[204] Knezevic I, Griffiths E, Reigel F, et al. Thimerosal in vaccines: a regulatory perspective. WHO Consultation, Geneva, 15–16 April 2002. Vaccine 2004;22:1836–41.

[205] Blaxill MF, Redwood L, Bernard S. Thimerosal and autism? A plausible hypothesis that should not be dismissed. Med Hypotheses 2004;62(5):788–94.

[206] SafeMinds. SafeMinds urges advisory committee for immunization practices to state a preference for thimerosal-free vaccines. July 5, 2006. Available at: http://www.SafeMinds.org. Accessed August 2006.

[207] Hoover AW, Goldwater LJ. Absorption and excretion of mercury in man. X. dental amalgams as a source of urinary mercury. Arch Environ Health 1966;12(4):506–8.

[208] Lorscheider FL, Vimy MJ, Summers AO. Mercury exposure from "silver" tooth fillings: emerging evidence questions a traditional dental paradigm [see comment]. FASEB J 1995;9(7):504–8.

[209] Berglund A. Estimation by a 24-hour study of the daily dose of intra-oral mercury vapor inhaled after release from dental amalgam [see comment]. J Dent Res 1990;69(10): 1646–51.

[210] Langworth S, Kolbeck KG, Akesson A. Mercury exposure from dental fillings. II. release and absorption. Swed Dent J 1988;12(1–2):71–2.

[211] Oskarsson A, Schultz A, Skerfving S, et al. Total and inorganic mercury in breast milk in relation to fish consumption and amalgam in lactating women. Arch Environ Health 1996; 51(3):234–41.

[212] Snapp KR, Boyer DB, Peterson LC, et al. The contribution of dental amalgam to mercury in blood. J Dent Res 1989;68(5):780–5.

[213] Abraham JE, Svare CW, Frank CW. The effect of dental amalgam restorations on blood mercury levels. J Dent Res 1984;63(1):71–3.

[214] Sallsten G, Thoren J, Barregard L, et al. Long-term use of nicotine chewing gum and mercury exposure from dental amalgam fillings. J Dent Res 1996;75(1):594–8.

[215] Gay DD, Cox RD, Reinhardt JW. Chewing releases mercury from fillings. Lancet 1979; 1(8123):985–6.

[216] Berdouses E, Vaidyanathan TK, Dastane A, et al. Mercury release from dental amalgams: an in vitro study under controlled chewing and brushing in an artificial mouth. J Dent Res 1995;74(5):1185–93.

[217] Ozuah PO, Lesser MS, Woods JS, et al. Mercury exposure in an urban pediatric population. Ambul Pediatr 2003;3(1):24–6.

[218] Endo T, Nakaya S, Kimura R, et al. Gastrointestinal absorption of inorganic mercuric compounds in vivo and in situ. Toxicol Appl Pharmacol 1984;74(2):223–9.
[219] Vimy MJ, Lorscheider FL. Intra-oral air mercury released from dental amalgam. J Dent Res 1985;64(8):1069–71.
[220] Reinhardt JW, Boyer DB, Svare CW, et al. Exhaled mercury following removal and insertion of amalgam restorations. J Prosthet Dent 1983;49(5):652–6.
[221] Levy M, Schwartz S, Dijak M, et al. Childhood urine mercury excretion: dental amalgam and fish consumption as exposure factors. Environ Res 2004;94(3):283–90.
[222] Ahlqwist M, Bengtsson C, Lapidus L, et al. Serum mercury concentration in relation to survival, symptoms, and diseases: results from the prospective population study of women in Gothenburg, Sweden. Acta Odontol Scand 1999;57(3):168–74.
[223] Bjorkman L, Pedersen NL, Lichtenstein P. Physical and mental health related to dental amalgam fillings in Swedish twins. Community Dent Oral Epidemiol 1996;24(4): 260–7.
[224] Saxe SR, Snowdon DA, Wekstein MW, et al. Dental amalgam and cognitive function in older women: findings from the Nun Study. J Am Dent Assoc 1995;126(11):1495–501.
[225] Factor-Litvak P, Hasselgren G, Jacobs D, et al. Mercury derived from dental amalgams and neuropsychologic function. Environ Health Perspect 2003;111(5):719–23.
[226] US Public Health Service CtCEHaRP, Subcommittee on risk management. Dental amalgam: a scientific review and recommended public health service strategy for research, education, and regulation. Washington, DC: US Public Health Service; 1993.
[227] DeRouen TA, Leroux BG, Martin MD, et al. Issues in design and analysis of a randomized clinical trial to assess the safety of dental amalgam restorations in children. Control Clin Trials 2002;23(3):301–20.
[228] DeRouen TA, Martin MD, Leroux BG, et al. Neurobehavioral effects of dental amalgam in children: a randomized clinical trial [see comment]. JAMA 2006;295(15):1784–92.
[229] Bellinger DC, Trachtenberg F, Barregard L, et al. Neuropsychological and renal effects of dental amalgam in children: a randomized clinical trial [see comment]. JAMA 2006;295(15): 1775–83.
[230] Children's Amalgam Trial Study G. The Children's Amalgam Trial: design and methods. Control Clin Trials 2003;24(6):795–814.
[231] Needleman HL. Mercury in dental amalgam—a neurotoxic risk? [comment] JAMA 2006; 295(15):1835–6.
[232] Catsakis LH, Sulica VI. Allergy to silver amalgams. Oral Surg 1978;46:371–5.
[233] Duxbury AJ, Ead RD, McMurrough S, et al. Allergy to mercury in dental amalgam. Br Dent J 1982;152:47–50.
[234] Dorea JG. Mercury and lead during breast-feeding. Br J Nutr 2004;92(1):21–40.
[235] Anderson HA, Wolff MS. Environmental contaminants in human milk. J Expo Anal Environ Epidemiol 2000;10(6 Pt 2):755–60.
[236] Vimy MJ, Hooper DE, King WW, et al. Mercury from maternal "silver" tooth fillings in sheep and human breast milk. A source of neonatal exposure. Biol Trace Elem Res 1997; 56(2):143–52.
[237] Lindow SW, Knight R, Batty J, et al. Maternal and neonatal hair mercury concentrations: the effect of dental amalgam. BJOG 2003;110(3):287–91.
[238] Drasch G, Aigner S, Roider G, et al. Mercury in human colostrum and early breast milk. Its dependence on dental amalgam and other factors. J Trace Elem Med Biol 1998;12(1): 23–7.
[239] Drexler H, Schaller KH. The mercury concentration in breast milk resulting from amalgam fillings and dietary habits. Environ Res 1998;77(2):124–9.
[240] Stoz F, Aicham P, Jovanovic S, et al. [Effects of new dental amalgam fillings in pregnancy on Hg concentration in mother and child. With consideration for possible interactions between amalgam and precious metals]. Zentralblatt fur Gynakologie 1995;117(1):45–50 [in German].

[241] Klemann D, Weinhold J, Strubelt O, et al. [Effects of amalgam fillings on the mercury concentrations in amniotic fluid and breast milk]. Deutsche Zahnarztliche Zeitschrift 1990; 45(3):142–5 [in German].

[242] Grandjean P, Weihe P, Needham LL, et al. Relation of a seafood diet to mercury, selenium, arsenic, and polychlorinated biphenyl and other organochlorine concentrations in human milk. Environ Res 1995;71(1):29–38.

[243] da Costa SL, Malm O, Dorea JG. Breast-milk mercury concentrations and amalgam surface in mothers from Brasilia, Brazil. Biol Trace Elem Res 2005;106(2):145–51.

[244] WHO (World Health Organization). Inorganic mercury. Volume 118 of Environmental Health Criteria. International Programme on Chemical Safety. Geneva: World Health Organization, 1991.

[245] Sandborgh-Englund G, Einarsson C, Sandstrom M, et al. Gastrointestinal absorption of metallic mercury. Arch Environ Health 2004;59(9):449–54.

[246] Bjornberg KA, Vahter M, Berglund B, et al. Transport of methylmercury and inorganic mercury to the fetus and breast-fed infant. Environ Health Perspect 2005;113(10):1381–5.

[247] Juszkiewicz T, Szprengier T, Radomanski T. [Mercury content of human milk]. Pol Tyg Lek 1975;30(9):365–6 [in Polish].

[248] Mata L, Sanchez L, Calvo M. Interaction of mercury with human and bovine milk proteins. Biosci Biotechnol Biochem 1997;61(10):1641–5.

[249] Dorea JG, Horner MR, Campanate ML. Longitudinal study of major milk constituents from two socioeconomic groups of mothers in Brazil. Nutr Rep Int 1984;29:699–710.

[250] Smith KM, Sahyoun NR. Fish consumption: recommendations versus advisories, can they be reconciled? Nutr Rev 2005;63(2):39–46.

[251] US Food and Drug Administration. Center for Food Safety and Applied Nutrition. Office of Seafood. Mercury levels in seafood species. Available at: http://vm.cfsan.fda.gov/~frf/sea-mehg.html. Accessed January 7, 2005.

[252] U.S. Environmental Protection Agency. Federal register environmental documents. Reference dose for methylmercury. Available at: http://www.epa.gov/fedrgstr/EPA-MEETINGS/2000/October/Day-30/m27781.html. Accessed January 7, 2005.

[253] U.S. Department of Health and Human Services and U.S. Environmental Protection Agency. FDA and EPA announce the revised consumer advisory on methylmercury in fish. Available at: http://www.fda.gov/bbs/topics/news/2004/NEW01038.html. Accessed January 6, 2005.

[254] Institute of Medicine. Committee on Nutrient Relationships in Seafood. Seafood choices: balancing benefits and risks. Available at: http://www.nap.edu. Accessed July 2006.

ELSEVIER
SAUNDERS

Pediatr Clin N Am
54 (2007) 271–294

PEDIATRIC CLINICS

OF NORTH AMERICA

Update on the Clinical Management of Childhood Lead Poisoning

Alan D. Woolf, MD, MPH[a,b,c,*],
Rose Goldman, MD, MPH[a,b,d,e],
David C. Bellinger, PhD, MSc[a,b,e,f]

[a]*Harvard Medical School, 25 Shattuck Street Boston, MA 02115, USA*
[b]*New England Pediatric Environmental Health Subspecialty Unit, Children's Hospital,
300 Longwood Avenue, Boston, MA 02115, USA*
[c]*Division of General Pediatrics, Children's Hospital, 300 Longwood Avenue,
Boston, MA 02115, USA*
[d]*Division of Occupational & Environmental Medicine, Cambridge Hospital,
1493 Cambridge Street, Cambridge, MA 02138, USA*
[e]*Department of Environmental Health, Harvard School of Public Health,
677 Huntington Avenue, Boston, MA 02115, USA*
[f]*Department of Neurology, Children's Hospital Boston, 300 Longwood Avenue,
Boston, MA 02115, USA*

The clinical landscape with respect to childhood lead poisoning is changing. The definition of childhood plumbism has been revised downwards four times within the past 45 years as more has been learned about subtle but important neurologic toxicity of chronic exposure to even relatively low body burdens. Public health prevention measures, such as removal of lead from gasoline, have resulted in declines in the number of children in the United States who have blood lead concentrations greater than 10 μg/dL from 77.8% in 1980 to 1.6% by 2002. Special groups of children, however, such as the economically disadvantaged, recent immigrants, and children who have developmental delays, are at a disproportionately higher risk of lead contamination. An estimated 24 million housing units in the United States still have lead paint hazards and need abatement.

This work was supported in part by a grant from the Agency for Toxic Substances and Disease Registry Superfund Reconciliation & Reclamation Act, administered through the Association of Occupational and Environmental Clinics Association, Washington, DC.

* Corresponding author. Division of General Pediatrics, Children's Hospital Boston, 300 Longwood Avenue, Boston, MA 02115.

E-mail address: alan.woolf@childrens.harvard.edu (A.D. Woolf).

Lingering cognitive, behavioral, and other adverse effects of lead poisoning may follow the victims throughout childhood and into adolescence and adulthood, exacting an enormous human toll on society in terms of lost productivity, special educational needs, and other medical as well as economic and social consequences. It is incumbent on health professionals to remain vigilant for cases of childhood lead poisoning by screening high-risk children, counseling families regarding effective lead poisoning prevention measures, and introducing parents to strategies that positively influence children's diets, behaviors, and the safety of their homes. To spare a new generation the unfortunate legacy of injury from exposure to this toxic metal, pediatricians also must act as advocates for the right of children to live in a lead-safe environment.

Epidemiology of childhood lead poisoning

Although progress in the reduction of environmental sources of lead in the United States has been dramatic during the past 30 years, childhood lead poisoning continues to challenge the pediatric health care provider in many communities. The annual cost of the health effects of lead exposure in the United States has been estimated at $43.5 billion, which is much higher than that associated with other environmental toxins [1]. Although lead has long been banned in house paint, gasoline, and other sources, such as metal cans and indoor plumbing solder, it is still present in older housing. A nationally representative survey conducted from 1998 to 2000 estimated that 38 million housing units in the United States had lead-based paint (down from 64 million in 1990), with an estimated 24 million units having significant lead paint hazards [2]. Housing in the Northeast and Midwest had twice the prevalence of lead contamination hazards as housing in the South and West, with a disproportionately higher number of low-income units affected.

In addition, an estimated 4 to 5 million tons of lead has been deposited in the soil in the United States from the use of gasoline-fueled motor vehicles [3]. The ingestion of lead-containing soil and dust by hand-to-mouth behaviors during outside play in contaminated external environments is generally underappreciated. The pattern of fluctuation in children's blood lead levels has been correlated in part with seasonal higher temperatures, lower soil moisture content, and the resuspension and dispersal of exterior dust [4].

National Health and Nutrition Examination Survey trends

The Centers for Disease Control and Prevention (CDC), conducting three iterations of the National Health and Nutrition Examination Survey (NHANES) from 1976 to 1980, 1991 to 1994, and 1999 to 2002, has documented a steady decline in the number of children 1 to 5 years old in the United States with blood lead levels greater than 10 μg/dL, from 77.8% to 4.4% to 1.6%, respectively [5]. Approximately 310,000 children (90% confidence interval, 275,000–810,000) are still affected by elevated lead levels.

This dramatic decline in blood lead levels has resulted in significant benefits in improved health and productivity, with the benefit in averted health costs estimated at $312 billion [6,7]. Nonetheless, recent studies suggest that there is no threshold for injury from absorbed lead in children, and blood lead levels less than 10 μg/dL have been correlated with lowered IQ scores [8,9].

Disparities in childhood lead poisoning

Children's risk for lead poisoning correlates with their ability to walk, their hand-to-mouth behaviors, and their oral exploratory habits. Typically peak blood lead levels occur by 18 to 30 months of age and then decline gradually through the rest of the toddler and school-aged years. There are important disparities in who has elevated lead levels in the United States, with poor urban children of color being disproportionately affected by high body lead burdens. Children living in poverty and receiving Medicaid benefits, whose parents are more likely to rent housing in districts where the housing is of lower value, had disproportionately higher blood lead levels than others [5,10,11].

Children who have developmental delays

Children who have persistent pica behaviors are at high risk for continued lead exposure well into the school-aged years. Those children include those who have autistic spectrum disorder (ASD), pervasive developmental delays (PDD), and other developmental delays. Neurotoxicity attributable to childhood lead poisoning is a comorbidity for many children who have ASD/PDD. Previous studies have theorized that a subset of children who have autism (ie, those who continue to demonstrate pica behaviors for nonfood objects throughout childhood) are at a high risk for plumbism. Almost 30 years ago, Cohen and colleagues [12] compared blood lead concentrations in 18 autistic children with levels in 16 children who had childhood psychosis and 10 normal controls and found levels to be significantly higher, affecting a wider age range and all social classes, in the children who had autism than the control groups. Accardo and colleagues [13] reported six cases of infantile autism and associated lead poisoning and postulated that the pica behaviors preceded and were causally related to the lead poisoning. There is only a single case report of an apparent improvement in repetitive behaviors and hyperactivity in a 4-year-old child who had autism and plumbism after he was treated with dimercaptosuccinic acid (DMSA) chelation [14]. The unique characteristics of children who have both autism and lead poisoning were described by Shannon and Graef [15] in a study of 17 children who had PDD and elevated lead levels compared with 30 controls treated for plumbism who had normal development. Those who had PDD presented with de novo lead poisoning at a later age (mean age, 46.5 versus 14.1 months) and had re-exposures later into childhood than did controls. Currently many pediatric practitioners do not screen children beyond the age of 3 years, so there may be a significant number of unrecognized cases among the cohort of children who have developmental disorders.

International adoption

More families in the United States are adopting children from foreign countries, children who may not have had access to health care services in their home countries and who may have been living in homes contaminated by lead-containing paint, plaster, cribs, furniture, or drinking water. In the medical assessment of such children, the discovery of an elevated blood lead level is common. Infants and young children who are international adoptees should be screened for lead poisoning on their arrival in the United States, and appropriate prevention and treatment measures should be undertaken if levels are found to be elevated. Homes into which young children are being adopted also should be assessed for lead contamination hazards.

Immigrant children

Children who emigrate to the United States from other countries (eg, from Asia, Africa or Eastern Europe) may have acquired lead poisoning in their home countries if they come from poverty-stricken households where dilapidated housing, poor industrial and environmental controls, continued use of leaded gasoline, and/or squalid living conditions expose the children to lead contamination.

Sources of lead exposure

Lead is found in paint chips, plaster, and dust in older, deteriorating housing built before the 1970s and often is spread by interior renovations. Most young children are poisoned by the ingestion of lead-containing dust from hand-to-mouth behaviors. Lead from chipping and peeling exterior house paint or from power sanding the exteriors of contaminated buildings during renovation also contaminates outdoor soils. Residual soil deposits may exist from the previous use of leaded gasoline or lead arsenate pesticides, from contaminated landfills and previous industrial concerns, or from proximity to industrial emissions from foundries, smelters, or other industrial users. Sanding, demolition, or renovation of nearby contaminated buildings may introduce new sources of lead into nearby environments. Lead has been discovered in many unexpected products, from eye cosmetics to crayons, crafts supplies, and children's toys [16]. Box 1 summarizes these ubiquitous sources of lead contamination.

Lead in ethnic remedies

Significant amounts of lead have been reported as a contaminant or an intentional adulterant in some herbs and ethnic remedies, such as Ayurvedic herbal products [17]. Severe lead poisoning was diagnosed in the preterm

---

Box 1. Sources of childhood lead poisoning

Environmental sources
Antique toys, cribs, or furniture
Contaminated foodstuffs: homegrown vegetables, imported
  spices, calcium supplements, flour
Cosmetics (eg, kohl, surma, ceruse)
Crafts (ceramic glazes, paint pigments, stained glass–making
  materials)
Decorative exterior home features (eg, "pewter-look" fencing)
Drinking water (especially first morning draw, hot water)
Dust
Folk remedies (eg, litarigio, greta, azarcon, alkohl, bali bali, coral,
  ghasard, liga, pay-loo-ah, reuda)
Herbal products
Imported toys, crayons
Imported ceramics or pewter
Imported soldered pots, kettles
Methamphetamine
Moonshine whiskey
Paint
Plaster, putty
Soil

Exposures from activities
Burning painted wood
Hobbies (eg, target shooting, stained glass making, glazing
  pottery)
Home renovation
Occupations (eg, auto repair, mining, smelting, demolition,
  battery manufacture, remodeling, construction, painting, pipe
  fitting, plumbing, shipbuilding, welding, bridge reconstruction,
  firing range instructors)

In utero exposures: maternal lead poisoning
Occupational exposures (see above)
Hobbies (see above)
Pica/geophagia
Herbal products
Dietary supplements

---

infant born to a 24-year-old Indian woman who had used lead- and mercury-contaminated medicinal tablets before and during her pregnancy [18]. Lead poisoning also has been associated with Hispanic folk remedies, such as "litargirio," a peach-colored powder that can contain up to 79%

lead monoxide [19] and lead oxide– and lead tetroxide–containing "greta" [20] and "azarcon" [21], Mexican compounds used to treat abdominal conditions. Indian folk remedies [22] and folk remedies used by Hmong Vietnamese [23] to treat their children also have resulted in lead poisoning. Other examples are given in Box 1.

Lead in spices, infant milk, and foodstuffs

The New England Pediatric Environmental Health Specialty Unit (PEHSU) located in Boston treated two families, one from India and one from the Republic of Georgia, in whom all of the family members suffered lead poisoning from bulk spices they had purchased from street vendors in their home countries and had brought into the United States to be used in their daily meals. In the Georgian family, the 4-year-old boy had a blood lead level of 31 µg/dL after eating meals containing swanuri marili (Pb 2040 ppm) and kharchos suneli (Pb 23,100 ppm) for several months [24]. Lead also has been found as a contaminant of Middle Eastern flour [25], calcium supplements [26], and imported candies [27]. The use of lead-containing or lead-soldered cooking pans, kettles, and glazed pottery to serve food or beverages to the family also may represent an overlooked hazard in the home. The New England PEHSU recorded a case of lead poisoning in a 4-month-old infant (peak blood lead level, 46 µg/dL) whose parents routinely reconstituted his infant formula with water previously boiled in an imported, lead-soldered samovar [28]. Two young children suffered lead poisoning, and one died, after drinking apple juice stored in lead-glazed earthenware jugs [29].

Lactating women can mobilize lead from bony stores and increase their own exposure as well as that of their unborn infant, although a recent study of 310 lactating women determined that breast milk lead levels, although correlating with infant blood lead levels, were fairly low (0.21–8.0 ugm/L), even among women who themselves had significant blood lead levels (geometric mean 8.4 µm/dL) [30].

Pregnant women who are exposed to lead occupationally or from other sources may put the fetus at high risk of lead accumulation, with a variety of consequent injuries reflected in pregnancy outcomes, including poor postnatal growth and development.

Pathophysiology of plumbism

Children are at higher risk for lead poisoning than adults for several reasons. They absorb a higher proportion of ingested lead, distribute more of it to water-soluble reservoirs in soft tissues rather than bone, have an immature blood–brain barrier resulting in increased penetration of lead into the central nervous system, and have developing body systems (blood, bone, immune, kidney, brain, and nervous system) that are more susceptible to injury at the cellular level. Children are more likely to have iron deficiency, a comorbidity of lead poisoning, that enhances lead's absorption, changes its kinetics, and works synergistically to increase the vulnerability of children to developmental delays.

Primary injury

Lead neurotoxicity may derive from two different basic mechanisms: interference with neurotransmission at the synapse and interference with cell adhesion molecules, causing disruption in cellular migration during critical periods of central nervous system development. In many organ systems, lead can interfere with a variety of enzyme systems and the cell's synthetic functions. For example, the synthesis of heme in red blood cells is dependent on rate-limiting enzymes such as ferrochetalase and delta amino levulinic acid dehydratase, both of which are inhibited early in lead poisoning, resulting in the microcytic, hypochromic anemia seen in affected children. There is new evidence in mice that, as an immunotoxicant, lead can disrupt T-cell function [31]. Lead also is toxic to osteoblasts, induces chondrogenesis, inhibits new bone vascularization, and affects mineralization of cartilage. It can cause impaired 1-alpha hydroxylation of cholecalciferol (the precursor to active vitamin D) in the kidneys. Such cellular effects have clinical implications, promoting osteopenia, osteoporosis, and defective hydroxyapatite lattice formation during skeletal bone growth or fracture healing [32].

Secondary health effects

Childhood lead poisoning causes a variety of neurologic injuries, including cognitive losses, aggression, hyperactivity, impulsivity, inattention, and learning failure. It may have some influence on physical growth and reproductive efficiency. It also may be an antecedent condition leading to both hypertension and chronic renal dysfunction in adults [33–36].

Magnitude of lead-associated decline in neurodevelopmental function

The endpoint for which the most data are available to use in quantifying the likely magnitude of the impact of lead on neurodevelopment is IQ, although recognition is widespread, and growing, that IQ might not be the most sensitive endpoint. Several meta-analyses of the available observational epidemiologic studies indicate that children's IQ scores decline two to three points per 10-μg/dL increase in blood lead level [37,38]. This estimate of the slope of the dose–effect relationship between blood lead level and IQ has important limitations, however. It pertains mostly to blood lead levels in the range of 10 to 30 μg/dL. Most importantly, it assumes that the functional form of the dose–effect relationship is linear, that is, that the IQ decline for each 1-μg/dL increase in blood lead level is constant across the entire range of levels. Several recent studies, including a pooled analysis of seven prospective studies involving 1333 children, suggest, somewhat surprisingly, that the rate of decline in IQ scores might be greater at blood lead levels below 10 μg/dL than at levels higher than 10 μg/dL [8,9,39–41]. In the pooled analysis, the log-linear model, the functional form that best described the data, predicted a 9.2-point decline in IQ over the range of less than 1 to 30 μg/dL [41]. Two thirds of the decline (6.2 points) was predicted to occur in the blood lead range of less than 1 to 9.9 μg/dL, with an additional 1.9-point decline between 10 and 19.9 μg/dL and a 1.1-point decline between 20 and 30 μg/dL. A plausible biologic mechanism for such a supralinear relationship has not been identified but presumably would involve a lead-sensitive pathway that is saturated rapidly at blood lead levels less than 10 μg/dL and other, less rapidly saturated pathways that are involved at blood lead levels greater than 10 μg/dL.

Nature of lead-associated neurodevelopmental injuries

There is no single neurodevelopmental finding that unequivocally identifies a child as having an elevated blood lead level, nor does there seem to be a group of findings that, in aggregate, define a "signature" injury. Lead-associated deficits have been reported in almost all major domains of function, including verbal IQ, performance IQ, academic skills such as reading and mathematics, visual–spatial skills, problem-solving skills, executive functions, fine and gross motor skills, memory, and language skills. It would be surprising if the way in which neurodevelopmental toxicity is expressed does not depend on cohort characteristics such as age at exposure, coexposures to other neurotoxicants, nutritional status, genotype, and the characteristics of the home environment. Experimental studies in rodents show that being reared in a stimulating environment can reduce the severity of lead-associated deficits [42], whereas being reared in a stressful environment can exacerbate them [43]. Recent data have challenged, to some extent, the traditional view that children are at greatest risk in the first few postnatal years. In some studies of outcomes at school age, it was concurrent blood level, rather than the levels measured in early childhood, that bore the strongest association with IQ [44–46].

Although increased lead burdens consistently have been shown to increase the risk of behaviors linked to the inattentive subtype of attention-deficit hyperactivity disorder (distractibility, disorganization, daydreaming), to date conclusive evidence that lead causes attention-deficit hyperactivity disorder is lacking. On the other hand, to date no study has provided an adequate test of this hypothesis. In Rhesus monkeys, lead exposure decreases social play and increases self-stimulatory behavior, interfering with peer relationships [47]. Recently, several studies have shown that higher blood or bone lead levels are associated with antisocial behaviors and poor educational outcomes in children and adolescents [48–52]. Higher exposure to lead during the second trimester of pregnancy may be associated with an increased risk of schizophrenia in children [53].

The results of long-running prospective studies provide little reason to expect that lead-associated neurodevelopmental deficits associated with postnatal exposure resolve over time [54]. Chelation therapy has not yet been shown to be effective in preventing or reversing cognitive deficits associated with blood lead levels between 20 and 44 μg/dL [55,56]. These data thus suggest that prevention of exposure is the most effective strategy for reducing lead-associated morbidity.

Case finding

Although erythrocyte protoporphyrin levels were used as a screening tool in the past, this test is not sensitive and has been replaced by the direct measurement of lead in whole blood. Clinicians are warned that, unless the finger is vigorously cleaned, a fingerstick blood lead test can give falsely high values from contaminating environmental dust. The venous blood lead level may be a more reliable route for testing.

The screening of children for possible lead poisoning targets high-risk groups according to the following CDC criteria:

Children living in housing constructed before 1978 containing paint or plaster in poor condition (ie, peeling, chipped, flaking paint, broken or crumbling plaster)

Children living near lead-smelting or -processing plants, battery recycling facilities, or other point sources of lead contamination

Children having parents or other household members who work in a lead-related occupation or have a lead-related hobby (eg, pottery, furniture refinishing)

Children whose siblings, playmates, or housemates have been recently diagnosed with lead poisoning

Children living in housing constructed before 1978 that is undergoing renovations likely to disrupt old plaster or painted surfaces

Although some states have adopted universal annual screening of preschool children 1 to 5 years old, others with limited resources have targeted screening programs to those children at the highest risk. The CDC has set a criterion of screening all Medicaid-eligible children and children living in high-risk communities (eg, those in which 12% or more of the children have blood lead levels ≥ 10 μg/dL). Screening of all international adoptees and immigrant children from areas known to have lead-contaminated environments seems prudent.

The risk of the fetus from maternal exposure to lead during pregnancy is substantial, so that women engaged in occupations or crafts known to have a risk of lead contamination should be screened periodically with blood lead levels. Fetal accumulation of lead by simple diffusion across the placenta may be unidirectional, so that accumulations in fetal tissues exceed those in the mother. Interference with cellular differentiation and migration patterns at critical points in fetal development pose a risk of irreversible injury or stillbirth [57].

Assessment of childhood lead poisoning

The CDC has defined a blood lead level of 10 µg/dL as the threshold level of concern, although this level may be neither safe nor normal. When a blood lead level is found to be elevated to 10 µg/dL or higher, a complete assessment of the child's exposure risks is indicated. The blood lead level should be repeated at an appropriate time interval gauged to the height of the elevation before medical management is begun. This time period may range from 1 month later for blood lead levels of 10 to 19 µg/dL to a repeated test within 24 to 48 hours for a blood lead level of 45 µg/dL or higher (Table 1). Periodic rescreenings thereafter are performed at a frequency individualized to the child's case management.

A meticulous history is of paramount importance. Inquiry into the age and possible lead contamination of all the environments in which the child spends significant amounts of time should be undertaken. What is the age of the home? What landfills or commercial concerns are nearby? Have interior or exterior renovations taken place recently? Are the windows old? Are there bite marks on windowsills or furniture? Other sources of lead exposure, including water, toys, day care centers, and other novel sources outlined in this article, are important aspects of the pediatric history (see Box 1). Parental occupations and hobbies may reveal sources of lead contamination. The child's behaviors are important. Does the child have pica and oral exploratory behaviors? A dietary history and use of any dietary supplements are important. Does the family use filtered, bottled, or tap water for drinking? Are cooking utensils imported and soldered or glazed with lead? The family's attempt to control interior dust and their hand-washing habits should be queried.

A comprehensive physical examination, with an emphasis on the neurologic examination, is an essential aspect of the assessment. Parents may point out a child's irritability, insomnia, aggressiveness, lack of focus and attention, poor appetite, speech delays, or learning problems as harbingers of lead poisoning, although none of these is specific for the condition—all are seen in preschool children without elevated blood lead levels.

An abdominal radiograph may reveal recently ingested lead-laden paint chips or plaster that need to be evacuated to prevent further lead absorption. Long bone radiographs can show metaphyseal lead lines characteristic of chronic exposure.

A complete blood count and free erythrocyte protoporphyrin (FEP) or zinc-chelated protoporphyrin (ZPP) blood level may show the microcytic anemia typical of lead's interference with heme synthesis. Erythrocyte protoporphyrin levels can be elevated by an iron deficiency state as well as by early interference by lead in heme synthesis in the red blood cells. It can add information in the assessment of the chronicity of the poisoning as

Table 1
Recommendations for children who have confirmed (venous) elevated blood lead concentrations

Blood lead concentration	Recommendations
10–14 µg/dL	Lead education: dietary, environmental Follow-up blood lead monitoring within 1 month
15–19 µg/dL	Lead education: dietary, environmental Follow-up blood lead monitoring within 1 month Proceed according to actions for 20–44 µg/dL if follow-up blood lead concentration is in this range ≥3 months after the initial test or blood lead concentration increases
20–44 µg/dL	Lead education: dietary, environmental Follow-up blood lead monitoring within 1 week Complete history and physical examination Laboratory work: hemoglobin or hematocrit, iron status Environmental investigation Lead hazard reduction Neurodevelopmental monitoring Abdominal radiography (if particulate lead ingestion is suspected) with bowel decontamination if indicated
45–69 µg/dL	Lead education: dietary, environmental Follow-up blood lead monitoring within 48 hours Complete history and physical examination Laboratory work: hemoglobin or hematocrit, iron status, free erythrocyte protoporphyrin or zinc protoporphyrin Environmental investigation Lead hazard reduction Neurodevelopmental monitoring Abdominal radiography with bowel decontamination if indicated Chelation therapy
≥70 µg/dL	Hospitalize and commence chelation therapy Follow-up confirmation of blood lead level immediately Proceed according to actions for 45–69 µg/dL

Modified from Centers for Disease Control and Prevention. Managing elevated blood lead levels among young children: recommendations from the Advisory Committee on Childhood Lead Poisoning Prevention. Atlanta (GA): Centers for Disease Control & Prevention, 2002. Available at: www.cdc.gov/nceh/lead/Casemanagement/Casemanage.main/htm. Accessed June 11, 2006.

well as the presence of iron deficiency as a comorbidity. Screening the blood for adequacy of iron stores also might include serum iron and ferritin levels. An elevated FEP (or ZPP) in a child shown to be iron sufficient indicates a longer duration of exposure to lead, with a body burden that may be more refractory to successful chelation.

Management of childhood lead poisoning

The management of childhood lead poisoning relies on three sequential components: environmental abatement, nutritional supplementation, and pharmacologic therapy. The CDC defines a blood lead level of 10 µg/dL as the threshold level of concern, at which point active management of exposure to lead should be initiated, as reflected in Table 1. Recent studies, however, have documented harmful effects of lead on a child's cognitive development at even lower blood levels [8,9]. Acknowledging the uncertainty of a lower bound lead level associated with injury, individual pediatricians may wish to initiate close monitoring, dietary adjustments, and environmental controls for families of children who have a blood lead level lower than 10 μg/dL. At every level, a careful inspection and abatement of the child's home environment for sources of lead hazard is paramount in protecting the child from continued contamination.

The management of childhood lead poisoning should be multidisciplinary in approach and longitudinal in scope. Table 1 presents the CDC guidelines for different levels of intervention closely linked to blood lead concentrations.

Techniques for reducing environmental hazards

Currently, the major source of most childhood lead poisoning is dust and chips from deteriorating lead paint on interior surfaces. Before 1955, house paint could contain up to 50% lead. In 1971 the percentage was lowered to 1%, and in 1977 the Consumer Product Safety Commission limited the lead in most paints (except those for commercial or marine uses) to 0.06%. Although lead paint was removed from new use, an estimated 64 million homes in the United States still had lead-based paint by 1990. Beginning in 2003, the CDC and the US Department of Housing and Urban Development (HUD) required funded programs to develop formal plans to eliminate lead poisoning in their jurisdictions, which included eliminating lead paint hazards in housing [5,58]. State and local efforts have been encouraged and funded through HUD's Lead Based Control Grant Program (http://www.hud.gov/offices/lead/lhc/index.cfm), which provides grants of $1 million to $2.5 million to state and local governments for control of lead-based paint hazards in privately owned, low-income, owner-occupied and rental housing. The most recent NHANES survey of blood lead levels from 1999 to 2002 found a continued decline in the number of children with elevated blood lead levels that was thought to be partially attributable to the federal appropriations that helped decrease the number of homes with leaded paint to 38 million in 2000 [5]. Additionally, some states have instituted their own laws and regulations to control lead hazards to children.

What are specific measures to evaluate and control the lead hazard in the individual home? The Environmental Protection Agency (EPA) provides a number of useful booklets, most found on their Website (www.epa.gov/lead/pubs/leadpbed.htm#brochures), that describe assessment, temporary controls, and remediation. The first step is to determine if there actually is a potential lead hazard. Lead-based paint usually is not a hazard if it is in good condition and is not located on an impact or friction surface, such as a window

[59]. A checklist (http://www.epa.gov/lead/pubs/chancechecklist.pdf) of useful questions concerning environmental sources of lead is included.

Inspection

If environmental hazards in the home seem likely, the next step, ideally, would be to have the home inspected and tested by a certified professional. To locate a certified professional, one can call the National Lead Information Center at 1-800-424-LEAD or contact local sources provided on the EPA Website (www.epa.gov/lead). The EPA recommends testing for lead using portable X-ray fluorescence or by collecting paint chips for analysis [60]. The laboratory reports the amount of lead as weight of lead per weight of paint chip. The federal definition of lead-based paint is 0.5%, which is the same as 5000 µg/g or 5000 mg/kg or 5000 ppm. Test results also can be reported as milligrams per square centimeter; lead-based paint would be 1 mg/cm^2 or more. Key elements of the EPA's standards for residential housing include a dust lead hazard of less than 40 µg/square foot on floors and 250 µg/square foot on window sills. Soil lead hazards should be less than 400 ppm in play areas and less than 1200 ppm average for bare soil in the rest of the yard.

Temporary abatement

Immediate steps to reduce exposures temporarily include cleaning up any paint or plaster chips; cleaning floors, window frames, window sills, and other surfaces weekly with an all-purpose cleaner; thoroughly rinsing sponges and mop heads; washing children's hands often, especially before eating and nap/bed time; keeping play areas clean; keeping children from chewing window sills or other painted surfaces; and cleaning or removing shoes before entering the house after walking through lead-containing soil. Careful and frequent vacuuming using a high-efficiency particulate vacuum cleaner reduces household dust content without the risk of heating and vaporizing the lead in dust, which may occur with conventional vacuum cleaners. Other temporary measures include repairing damaged painted surfaces or using duct tape or contact paper to cover them entirely to create a physical barrier to access by the toddler. Covering bare soil in play areas outside with grass or mulch provides a barrier to exposure.

Environmental remediation

To remove lead hazards permanently, it is best to hire a certified lead abatement contractor who will use proper personal protective equipment and procedures. Abatement methods fall into three categories: (1) replacement: removing the building component, such as a window, and replacing it with a new one; (2) encapsulation: covering a lead-painted surface with a material that effectively prevents access to the lead paint and prevents

leaded dust from flaking off; (3) paint removal. Proper containment strategies and clean-up procedures during and after lead abatement are critical;
otherwise, the dwelling unit could be rendered more hazardous than before
abatement.

Role of diet in lead poisoning

Children who have dietary deficiencies in iron, calcium, vitamin C, or
zinc are more susceptible to injury from environmental sources of lead. In
large population studies, preschool urban children who had higher dietary
iron intake had lower blood lead levels [61]. Iron supplementation at 4 to
6 mg/kg/d is recommended for children who have lead poisoning and who
also have evidence of iron deficiency anemia. Iron-sufficient diets discourage
intestinal absorption from a common transport mechanism. Pica is associated with moderate iron deficiency, and this behavior also predisposes
children to ingestion of lead-contaminated nonfood items, thus compound-
ing an unhealthy pathway of vulnerability to lead poisoning.

Calcium competes with lead for enzyme systems and can inhibit its
absorption and bioavailability. Zinc deficiency also exacerbates the injury
caused by lead, because zinc competes with lead for binding sites on some
enzymes, such as delta aminolevulinic acid dehydratase. A diet replete
with zinc is protective and may inhibit some intestinal absorption of lead.
Phosphorus deficiency also increases lead absorption. Most American diets
have sufficient sources of both zinc and phosphorus.

Clinicians should routinely counsel families regarding optimal dietary
sources of iron, calcium, and vitamin C for young children at high risk for
lead poisoning. Box 2 shows some dietary sources of these essential nutrients.

Chelation

The first and primary treatment for lead poisoning is removal from exposure. In some circumstances, adding chelating medications that decrease
blood lead concentrations and increase urinary excretion of lead is also
indicated. Box 3 includes brief profiles of each of the chelation agents
commonly used in the management of lead poisoning.

Dimercaprol

One of the first chelators was dimercaprol, also called "British anti-
Lewisite (BAL)," which was developed in 1946 as an antidote to German
arsenical war gases [62]. It was used to treat severe childhood lead poisoning
because it promoted the renal excretion through the formation of stable,
nontoxic, soluble lead chelates. Treatment with dimercaprol was seen as
beneficial because of the decline in death rate of children who had severe

---

Box 2. Dietary sources of iron and calcium

Sources of calcium
Milk, ice cream
Yoghurt
Cheese
Fish: sardines, anchovies, shrimp, trout, cod, mackerel, tuna,
    salmon, crab, lobster
Vegetables: cabbage, collards, kale, broccoli, spinach, bok choy,
    mustard greens
Fruits: oranges, pineapples, raisins, fortified orange juice
Almonds

Sources of iron
Meat: lean beef, veal, ham, pork, chicken, lamb
Cereal: iron fortified cereals, wheat germ
Fish: clams, mussels, oysters, tuna, trout, cod, sardines, others
Fruits: dried fruits (apricots, raisins, prunes, dates)
Eggs
Liver
Vegetables (only fair sources): spinach, collard greens, lentils,
    peas, beans, peanut butter

Sources of vitamin C
Fruits: grapefruit, oranges, cantaloupe, strawberries, juices
Vegetables: broccoli, green peppers, greens

---

lead encephalopathy: from a rate of about 65% in the 1940s (before use of chelators) to less than 5% among similar cases treated with chelators in the 1960s [63–66]. Dimercaprol, which is dissolved in peanut oil for deep intramuscular injection, is associated with a high incidence of adverse effects, which include nausea and vomiting, hypertension, prolongation of the partial thromboplastin time, fever, rashes, and pain at the injection site. It is contraindicated in persons who have peanut allergy or hepatic insufficiency and may cause hemolysis in individuals who have glucose-6-phosphatase deficiency. Iron therapy needs to be discontinued because dimercaprol and iron form a complex that causes vomiting.

Calcium disodium ethylenediaminetetraacacetate

Another chelating agent, calcium disodium ethylenediaminetetraacacetate (CaNa2 EDTA) was introduced in the early 1950s. It increases the urinary excretion of lead 20-fold to 50-fold through the formation of nonionizing salts. CaNa2EDTA removes lead from the extracellular compartment only, because it does not enter cells. WARNING: Some hospitals still

---

Box 3. Medicines used to treat childhood lead poisoning

2.3-dimercaptopropanol; British anti-Lewisite, dimercaprol
- Only given parenterally (intramuscular)
- Usual dose is 75 mg/m^2 body surface area every 4 hours
- Dissolved in peanut oil
- Contraindicated in children allergic to nuts or those who have glucose-6-phosphatase deficiency
- Can cause kidney dysfunction or zinc depletion

Calcium disodium ethyleneaminetetraacetate; edetate disodium calcium
- Only given parenterally (intramuscular or intravenous)
- Usual maximum dose is 1000 mg/m^2 body surface area/d
- Can cause kidney dysfunction

DMSA
- Comes as 100-mg capsules only
- Usual dose is one to four capsules, depending on child's weight, given three times daily for 5 days, then twice daily for 14 days
- Can cause elevated liver enzymes (uncommon) or skin rash (uncommon)
- Contraindicated in children who have hepatic insufficiency or those who have ongoing exposure to lead
- Capsules should be aired out before contents are mixed with food

D-penicillamine (3-mercapto-D-valine)
- Available as 250-mg capsule or tablet
- Do not give with milk, milk products, or iron supplements
- Give in juice or jelly on an empty stomach
- Often causes mild upset stomach or loose stools
- Can cause skin rash or zinc/iron depletion (common) or kidney or marrow dysfunction (uncommon)
- Usual dose is 10 to 15 mg/kg/d
- Contraindicated in children who have renal insufficiency or ongoing exposure to lead
- Capsules should be aired out before contents are mixed with food

---

stock the incorrect EDTA salt. It is crucial that the calcium disodium salt be used, because the disodium EDTA salt alone binds calcium and can cause severe hypocalcemia and possible death. CaNa2EDTA can be given intravenously or intramuscularly, usually for 5 days per chelation period.

The major side effects include local reaction at the injection sites, fever, calcium abnormalities, renal dysfunction, and excretion of essential minerals. Several case series demonstrated the increased effectiveness and decreased toxicity of CaNa2EDTA when used as single treatment for severe lead poisoning [66]. A small, randomized, clinical trial in the 1960s showed that a two-drug regimen of dimercaprol and CaNa2EDTA resulted in a more rapid decline in blood lead concentration and greater urinary lead excretion [63].

Meso-2,3-dimercaptosuccinic acid

DMSA is a water-soluble analogue of dimercaprol that was approved by the Food and Drug Administration in 1991 for chelating children who have blood lead levels greater than 40 µg/dL. DMSA can be given orally, has less toxicity than CaNa2 EDTA, and causes less urinary loss of essential minerals. In case series, DMSA seemed to be slightly more effective than parenteral CaNa2EDTA in lowering blood lead concentrations in children who had blood lead levels of 50 to 69 µg/dL [67,68]. The most common adverse side effects listed on the label include abdominal distress, transient rash, elevated liver transaminase enzymes, and neutropenia. DMSA is supplied in 100-mg gelatin capsules that have a strong sulfur ("rotten egg") odor. It is administered orally for 5 days at a higher dose and 14 days at a lower dose.

D-penicillamine

Some clinicians use D-penicillamine, another oral chelating agent that is used in Wilson disease, for treating lead poisoning [69,70]. Its safety and efficacy have not been established for this use, however. When used for chelation of lead in young children, low doses (10-15 mg/kg/d) of oral D-penicillamine are recommended, and close monitoring of renal function and peripheral blood counts during therapy are also recommended. Allergic rashes, marrow suppression, and anaphylaxis are other adverse effects seen with this drug. The American Academy of Pediatrics' Committee on the Environment considers it to be a third-line drug for lead poisoning [71].

Approach to medical management

There are no randomized, clinical trials of lead poisoned children that have provided evidence that treatment with chelators improves clinical outcomes, particularly future cognitive development. Treatment regimens have been based largely on clinical judgment and case-based experiences.

For blood lead levels of 20 to 44 µg/dL: The American Academy of Pediatrics' Committee on Environmental Health states there are no data to support use of DMSA in children whose blood lead concentrations are less than 45 µg/dL if the goal is to improve cognition [71]. If chelation is attempted, first the lead hazard in the home should be reduced, and the child should be assessed to ensure no contraindications exist.

For blood lead level of 45 to 69 μg/dL: If exposure has been controlled, and there are no contraindications, treatment with DMSA should begin [71]. If the child cannot take DMSA, parenteral therapy with CaNa2EDTA and hospitalization is indicated. A pediatrician experienced in treating children who have lead poisoning should be consulted for managing children who have blood lead levels greater than 45 μg/dL and can be identified by contacting the regional PEHSU (www.aoec.org/pehsu.htm).

For blood lead levels greater than 70 μg/dL: Children who have symptoms of lead poisoning and blood concentrations higher than 70 ug/dL need parenteral therapy with CaNa2EDTA and hospitalization [71]. Some clinicians believe that dimercaprol should be administered first, followed by CaNa2EDTA plus dimercaprol. Others believe that, although combined dimercaprol and CaNa2EDTA may accelerate the decline in blood lead concentration, there has been little evidence to demonstrate that the addition of dimercaprol to CaNa2EDTA monotherapy improves clinical outcome, particularly if the blood lead level is less than 100 μg/dL [66].

Neuropsychologic testing and monitoring

In addition to the CDC-recommended environmental and medical evaluations, a child who has a blood lead level above 20 μg/dL also should undergo a neurodevelopment evaluation, and neurodevelopmental surveillance should continue to be an element of the long-range management plan. The apparent lag in adverse effect implies that the failure to identify deficits when a child is first discovered to have an elevated blood lead level should not result in a lowering of the guard. It is still possible that the child will express lead-associated deficits in the future. According to the case-management guidelines developed by the CDC [72], such deficits might not be apparent until the child is faced with the increased challenges associated with critical transitions in school:

- In the first grade when the key task is the acquisition of academic skills such as reading
- In the third or fourth grade when the key task shifts to using the basic academic skills to learn new material (ie, "reading to learn" versus "learning to read")
- In the middle school years, when children are expected to have developed the skills needed to plan, organize, and complete complex, multistep projects

Lead-associated deficits that are germane to all three transitions (academic skill acquisition, reading comprehension and math problem-solving, and executive functions) have been identified. Implicit in this recommendation is that neurodevelopmental surveillance should not end when a child reaches 6 years of age, the upper bound of the age range associated with the greatest risk of elevated exposure. Furthermore, the fact that a lead-exposed child successfully negotiated an earlier transition should not be interpreted as an indication that neurodevelopmental surveillance is not necessary around the time of future transitions, when new and different demands are imposed.

Special education needs

No data are available regarding nonmedical interventions that are especially helpful to children who have neurodevelopmental deficits secondary to an elevated blood lead level. Indeed, because the nature and severity of the deficits can be expected to vary depending on a child's specific characteristics and circumstances, a "one size fits all" intervention seems unlikely. Under these circumstances, the best approach probably is to develop interventions that address to a child's specific presenting problems, as is done routinely for children who have idiopathic learning difficulties. There seems no reason to conclude that identifying lead as the source of a problem would dictate a different approach to the problem than if the source were unknown. Nevertheless, this is an assumption.

Family education and prevention

Community-wide education campaigns can contribute to public awareness of the need for reductions in the risk of lead exposure. One such citywide demonstration project organized by the health department in Hartford, Connecticut, was successful in increasing the knowledge of lead hazards by parents of preschool children, who recalled specific segments of the advertising strategy [73].

Liaison to community-level agencies

Childhood lead poisoning often is accompanied by complex social, economic, housing, and legal issues for the family. Thus medical management must be integrated with community-based resources where they are available. Visiting nurses can assess the family's supports, can assist in the child's adherence to chelation medications and dietary supplements, and can counsel the parents on techniques to prevent lead poisoning in the home [74,75]. University-affiliated agricultural extension services may have programs for testing of residential water or soil for lead content. State public health agencies may provide education, outreach, and inspection services to prevent lead poisoning.

Advocacy for corollary legal, economic, and social issues

Legal advocates can counsel both landlords and tenants on their rights and obligations under state housing laws and can advise homeowners of their options for abatement. Banking and state health officials can advise homeowners and landlords of local, regional, and federal grants and loans to assist in the expenses of housing abatement and the tax credits that may be available. Social services can coordinate these community efforts and arrange emergency housing to protect the child from continuing exposure.

Primary prevention

As is the case with all childhood injuries and illnesses having environmental determinants, primary prevention is the cornerstone of lowering the societal burden of lead-associated health risks. Reduction in the smelting and commercial uses of lead by the substitution of safer alternative technologies and materials is to be encouraged. Vigilance to the many potential products that may contain lead and their interdiction before they enter the marketplace where they pose a risk to children is of obvious importance. The provision of a nurturing environment, in which children can grow and develop, with attention to learning enrichment, a healthy and varied diet, plenty of sleep, lead-free housing, and clean air, water, schools, and playgrounds, is the primary prevention measure that promotes the pediatrician's goals of a healthy and happy child.

Summary

There has been tremendous progress in the prevention of childhood lead poisoning during the past 30 years. The reduction in the population's geometric mean blood lead level has resulted in real human benefits, with gains in intelligence, productivity, and functional outcome. The potential health cost savings realized from such efforts for each cohort of 2-year-old children are estimated variously at between $110 and $312 billion [76,77]. Childhood lead poisoning in America still remains a serious public health challenge to pediatric health care providers, in terms of expanding the gains and extending the benefits of prevention and effective management to all children.

Appendix

Governmental agencies and nongovernmental organizations

Alliance for Healthy Homes; 202-543-1147; www.afhh.org.htm: provides additional information on residential lead contamination and how to safely remove it.

Coalition to End Childhood Lead Poisoning; 800-370-5323; www.leadsa fe.org.htm: provides information for parents regarding childhood lead poisoning and its treatment and prevention.

Centers for Disease Control & Prevention (CDC); www.cdc.gov/nceh/lead/grants/contacts/CLPPP%20Map.htm: provides state and local contacts for childhood lead poisoning prevention programs funded by the CDC.

Department of Housing & Human Development (HUD); www.hud.gov/offices/lead.htm: Office of Healthy Homes and Lead Hazard Control provides ability to track HUD's progress in the abatement of lead hazards in residences.

Environmental Protection Agency; www.epa.gov/lead.htm:
EPA Lead Awareness Program provides information on residential lead abatement.

EPA Safe Drinking Water Hotline; 1-800-426-4791

National Lead Information Center Hotline (1-800-LEAD-FYI) and Clearinghouse (1-800-424-LEAD): established by four Federal agencies (the EPA, CDC, HUD, and DOD) to provide the public and professional audiences with information in English or Spanish about lead poisoning and prevention.

National Lead Information Center
1019 19th St, NW, Suite 401
Washington, DC 20036
1-202-833-1071

Pediatric Environmental Health Subspecialty Units (PEHSU); www.aoec.org/pehsu.htm: Agency for Toxic Substances & Disease Registry (ATSDR)– and EPA-sponsored regional centers providing clinical evaluation and consultation regarding pediatric environmental health issues, including lead poisoning.

References

[1] Landrigan PJ, Schechter CB, Lipton JM, et al. Environmental pollutants and disease in American children: estimates of morbidity, mortality, and costs for lead poisoning, asthma, cancer, and developmental disabilities. Environ Health Perspect 2002;110:721–8.
[2] Jacobs DE, Clickner RP, Zhou JY, et al. Prevalence of lead-based paint hazards in U.S. housing. Environ Health Perspect 2002;110:A599–606.
[3] Mielke HW. Lead in New Orleans soils: new images in an urban environment. Environ Geochem Health 1994;16:123–8.
[4] Laidlaw MAS, Mielke HW, Filippelli GM, et al. Seasonality and children's blood lead levels: developing a predictive model using the climactic variables and blood lead data from Indianapolis, Indiana, Syracuse, New York, and New Orleans, Louisiana. Environ Health Perspect 2005;113:793–800.
[5] Centers for Disease Control and Prevention. Blood lead levels-United States, 1999–2002. MMWR Morb Mortal Wkly Rep 2005;54(20):513–6.
[6] Grosse SD, Matte TD, Schwartz J, et al. Economic gains resulting from the reduction in children's exposure to lead. Environ Health Perspect 2002;110:563–9.
[7] Rothenberg SJ, Rothenberg JC. Testing the dose-response specification in epidemiology: public health and policy consequences for lead. Environ Health Perspect 2005;113:1190–5.
[8] Canfield RI, Henderson CR, Cory-Slechta DA, et al. Intellectual impairment in children with blood lead concentrations below 10 micrograms per deciliter. N Engl J Med 2003;348:1517–26.
[9] Lanphear BP, Dietrich KN, Auinger P, et al. Cognitive deficits associated with blood lead levels <10 g/dL in US children and adolescents. Pub Health Rep 2000;115:521–9.

[10] Lanphear BP, Byrd RS, Auinger P, et al. Community characteristics associated with elevated blood lead levels in children. Pediatrics 1998;101:264–71.

[11] Agency for Toxic Substances & Disease Registry. Case studies in environmental medicine course SS3059: lead toxicity. Atlanta (GA): US Dept of Health and Human Services; 2000.

[12] Cohen DJ, Johnson WT, Caparulo BK. Pica and elevated blood lead level in autistic and atypical children. Am J Dis Child 1976;130:47–8.

[13] Accardo P, Whitman B, Caul J, et al. Autism and plumbism: a possible association. Clin Pediatr 1988;27:41–4.

[14] Eppright TD, Sanfacon JA, Horwitz EA. Attention deficit hyperactivity disorder, infantile autism, and elevated blood lead: a possible relationship. Mo Med 1996;93:136–8.

[15] Shannon M, Graef JW. Lead intoxication in children with pervasive developmental disorders. Clin Toxicol 1996;34:177–81.

[16] Van Arsdale JL, Leiker RD, Kohn M, et al. Lead poisoning from a toy necklace. Pediatrics 2004;114:1096–9.

[17] Saper RB, Kales SN, Paquin J, et al. Heavy metal content of Ayurvedic herbal medicine products. JAMA 2004;292:2868–72.

[18] Tait PA, Vora A, James S, et al. Severe congenital lead poisoning in a preterm infant due to a herbal remedy. Med J Aust 2002;177:193–5.

[19] Centers for Disease Control and Prevention. Lead poisoning associated with use of litargirio—Rhode Island, 2003. MMWR Morb Mortal Wkly Rep 2005;54:227–9.

[20] Centers for Disease Control and Prevention. Lead poisoning associated with use of traditional ethnic remedies—California, 1991–1992. MMWR Morb Mortal Wkly Rep 1993;42:521–4.

[21] Bose A, Vashistha K, O'Loughlin BJ. Azarcon por empacho–another cause of lead toxicity. Pediatrics 1983;72(1):106–8.

[22] Centers for Disease Control and Prevention. Lead poisoning associated death from Asian folk remedies—Florida. MMWR Morb Mortal Wkly Rep 1984;33:638, 643–5.

[23] Centers for Disease Control. Folk-remedy associated lead poisoning in Hmong children—Minnesota. MMWR Morb Mortal Wkly Rep 1983;32:555–6.

[24] Woolf AD, Woolf NT. Childhood lead poisoning in two families associated with spices used in food preparation. Pediatrics 2005;116:e314–8.

[25] Dona A, Dourakis S, Papapdimitropoulos B, et al. Flour contamination as a source of lead intoxication. Clin Toxicol 1999;37:109–12.

[26] Scelfo GM, Flegal AR. Lead in calcium supplements. Environ Health Perspect 2000;108:309–13.

[27] Lynch RA, Boatright DT, Moss SK. Lead-contaminated imported tamarind candy and children's blood lead levels. Pub Health Rep 2000;115:537–43.

[28] Shannon M. Lead poisoning from an unexpected source in a 4-month-old. Environ Health Perspect 1998;106(6):229–32.

[29] Klein M, Namer R, Harpur E, et al. Earthenware containers as a source of fatal lead poisoning. N Engl J Med 1970;283:669–72.

[30] Ettinger AS, Tellez-Rojo MM, Amarasiriwardena C, et al. Levels of lead in breast milk and their relation to maternal blood and bone lead levels at one month postpartum. Environ Health Perspect 2004;112:926–31.

[31] Farrer DG, Hueber SM, McCabe MJ. Lead enhances CD4$^+$ T cell proliferation indirectly by targeting antigen presenting cells and modulating antigen-specific interactions. Toxicol Appl Pharmacol 2005;207:125–37.

[32] Carmouche JJ, Puzas JE, Zhang X, et al. Lead exposure inhibits fracture healing and is associated with increased chondrogenesis, delay in cartilage mineralization, and a decrease in osteoprogenitor frequency. Environ Health Perspect 2005;113:749–55.

[33] Harlan WR, Landis R, Schmouder RL, et al. Blood lead and blood pressure—relationship in the adolescent and adult US population. JAMA 1985;253:530–4.

[34] Hu H, Aro A, Payton M, et al. The relationship of bone and blood lead to hypertension. JAMA 1996;275:1171–5.

[35] Kim R, Rotnitzky A, Sparrow D, et al. A longitudinal study of low-level lead exposure and impairment of renal function. JAMA 1996;275:1175–81.

[36] Gerr F, Letz R, Stikes L, et al. Association between bone lead concentration and blood pressure among young adults. Am J Ind Med 2002;42:98–106.

[37] Schwartz J. Low-level lead exposure and children's IQ: a meta-analysis and search for a threshold. Environ Res 1994;65:42–55.

[38] Pocock SJ, Smith M, Baghurst PA. Environmental lead and children's intelligence: a systematic review of the epidemiological evidence. Br Med J 1994;309:1189–97.

[39] Kordas K, Canfield RL, Lopez P, et al. Deficits in cognitive function and achievement in Mexican first-graders with low blood lead concentration. Environ Res 2006;100:371–86.

[40] Tellez-Rojo MM, Bellinger DC, Arroyo-Quiroz C, et al. Longitudinal associations between blood lead concentrations < 10 mcg/dL and neurobehavioral development in environmentally-exposed children in Mexico City. Pediatrics 2006;118:e323–30.

[41] Wasserman G, Graziano J, Roberts R. Low-level environmental lead exposure and children's intellectual function: an international pooled analysis. Environ Health Perspect 2005;113:894–9.

[42] Guilarte TR, Toscano CD, McGlothan JL, et al. Environmental enrichment reverses cognitive and molecular deficits induced by developmental lead exposure. Ann Neurol 2003;53:50–6.

[43] Virgolini MB, Chen K, Weston DD, et al. Interactions of chronic lead exposure and intermittent stress: consequences for brain catecholamine systems and associated behaviors and HPA axis function. Toxicol Sci 2005;87:469–82.

[44] Bellinger DC. Lead. Pediatrics 2004;113:1016–32.

[45] Dietrich KN, Berger OG, Succop PA, et al. The developmental consequences of low to moderate prenatal and postnatal lead exposure: intellectual attainment in the Cincinnati Lead Study Cohort following school entry. Neurotoxicol Teratol 1993;15:37–44.

[46] Chen A, Dietrich KN, Ware JH, et al. IQ and blood lead from 2 to 7 years of age: are the effects in older children the residual of high blood lead concentrations in 2-year-olds? Environ Health Perspect 2005;113:597–601.

[47] Lanphear BP, Hornung R, Khoury J, et al. Lead exposure and diet: differential effects on social development in the Rhesus monkey. Neurotoxicol Teratol 1991;13:429–40.

[48] Needleman HL, Reiss JA, Tobin MJ, et al. Bone lead levels and delinquent behavior. JAMA 1996;275:363–9.

[49] Needleman HL, McFarland C, Ness RB, et al. Bone lead levels in adjudicated delinquents. A case control study. Neurotoxicol Teratol 2002;24:711–7.

[50] Dietrich KN, Ris MD, Succop PA, et al. Early exposure to lead and juvenile delinquency. Neurotoxicol Teratol 2001;23:511–8.

[51] Stretesky PB, Lynch MJ. The relationship between lead exposure and homicide. Arch Pediatr Adolesc Med 2001;155:579–82.

[52] Fergusson DM, Horwood LJ, Lynskey MT. Early dentine lead levels and educational outcomes at 18 years. J Child Psychol Psychiatry 1997;38:471–8.

[53] Opler MGA, Brown AS, Graziano JH, et al. Prenatal lead exposure, δ-aminolevulinic acid, and schizophrenia. Environ Health Perspect 2004;112:548–52.

[54] Ris MD, Dietrich KN, Succop PA, et al. Early exposure to lead and neuropsychological outcome in adolescence. J Int Neuropsychol Soc 2004;10:261–70.

[55] Rogan WJ, Dietrich KN, Ware JH, et al. The effect of chelation therapy with Succimer on neuropsychological development in children exposed to lead. N Engl J Med 2001;344:1421–6.

[56] Dietrich KN, Ware JH, Salganik M, et al. Effect of chelation therapy on the neuropsychological and behavioral development of lead-exposed children after school entry. Pediatrics 2004;114:19–26.

[57] Kosnett MJ, Wedeen RP, Rothenberg SJ, et al. Recommendations for medical management of adult lead exposure. Environ Health Perspect 2007;115(3):463–71.

[58] President's Task Force on Environmental Health Risks and Safety Risks to Children. Eliminating childhood lead poisoning: a federal strategy targeting lead paint hazards. Washington, DC: US Department of Housing and Urban Development; 2000.

[59] Environmental Protection Agency. Protect your family from lead in your home. Washington, DC: Environmental Protection Agency; 2003.

[60] Environmental Protection Agency. Testing your home for lead: in paint, dust and soil. EPA publication #747-K-00-001. Washington, DC: Environmental Protection Agency; 2000.

[61] Hammad TA, Sexton M, Langenberg P. Relationship between blood lead and dietary iron intake in preschool children. Ann Epidemiol 1996;6:30–3.

[62] Hurwitz RL, Lee DA. Childhood lead poisoning: treatment Up To Date 2006;14:1.

[63] Chisolm JJ. The use of chelating agents in the treatment of acute and chronic lead intoxication in childhood. J Pediatr 1968;73:1–38.

[64] Coffin R, Phillips J, Staples WL, et al. Treatment of lead encephalopathy in children. J Pediatr 1966;69:198–206.

[65] Ennis JM, Harrision HE. Treatment of lead encephalopathy with BAL (2,3-dimercaptopropranol). Pediatrics 1950;5:853–68.

[66] Kosnett MJ. Lead. In: Brint JEA, editor. Critical care toxicology. Philadelphia: Elsevier Publishers; 2005. p. 821–36.

[67] Graziano JH. Role of 2,3-dimercaptosuccinic acid in the treatment of heavy metal poisoning. Med Toxicol 1986;1:155–62.

[68] Graziano JH, Lolacono NJ, Moulton T, et al. Controlled study of meso-2,3-dimercaptosuccinic acid for the management of childhood lead intoxicat ion. J Pediatr 1992;120:133–9.

[69] Shannon M, Graef JW, Lovejoy FHJ. Efficacy and toxicity of D-penicillamine in low-level lead poisoning. J Pediatr 1988;112:799–804.

[70] Shannon MW, Townsend MK. Adverse effects of reduced-dose d-penicillamine in children with mild to moderate lead poisoning. Ann Pharmacother 2000;34:15–8.

[71] Committee on Environmental Health, American Academy of Pediatrics. Lead exposure in children: prevention, detection, and management. Pediatrics 2005;116:1036–46.

[72] Centers for Disease Control and Prevention. Managing elevated blood lead levels in young children. Atlanta (GA): The U.S. Centers for Disease Control and Prevention; 2002.

[73] McLaughlin T, Humphries O, Nguyen T, et al. "Getting the Lead Out" in Hartford, Connecticut: a multifaceted lead-poisoning awareness campaign. Environ Health Perspect 2004;112:1–5.

[74] Brown MJ, McLaine P, Dixon S, et al. A randomized, community-based trial of home visiting to reduce blood lead levels in children. Pediatrics 2005;117:147–53.

[75] Woolf AD. Home visiting and childhood lead poisoning prevention. Pediatrics 2006;117:2328–30.

[76] Rothenberg SJ, Rothenberg JC. Testing the dose-response specification in epidemiology: public health and policy consequences for lead. Environ Health Perspect 2005;113:1190–5.

[77] Grosse SD, Matte TD, Schwartz J, et al. Economic gains resulting from reduction in children's exposure to lead. Environ Health Perspect 2002;110:563–9.

ELSEVIER
SAUNDERS

Pediatr Clin N Am
54 (2007) 295–307

PEDIATRIC CLINICS
OF NORTH AMERICA

Environments, Indoor Air Quality, and Children

Mark E. Anderson, MD[a],*, Gregory M. Bogdan, PhD[b]

[a]*Denver Health Affiliate, University of Colorado Denver and Health Sciences Center,*
777 Bannock Street, Mail Code 1911, Denver, CO 80204, USA
[b]*Denver Health Affiliate, University of Colorado Denver and Health Sciences Center,*
Rocky Mountain Poison and Drug Center, 777 Bannock Street, Mail Code 0180,
Denver, CO 80204, USA

Children in the United States spend most of their time indoors, be this time spent at home or at school, and consideration of the quality of the indoor air is at least as important as consideration of outdoor air quality. Surprisingly little regulation occurs over the indoor environments in which children find themselves, with two exceptions: water quality (ie, lead and other toxicants) and asbestos. Rather, the approach taken by the US Environmental Protection Agency (EPA) is to encourage voluntary cooperation in programs such as the Healthy School Environments Assessment Tool. The EPA provides information and suggestions regarding the management of several indoor air problems including Environmental Tobacco Smoke (ETS), biologic contaminants such as mold and mildew, carbon monoxide (CO), lead, pesticides, radon, and others.

Pediatricians may find themselves poorly prepared to field questions from anxious parents when environmental health questions arise. Residency programs focus little attention on environmental health, and this area is, indeed, one in which "Internet science" informs more than traditional science, with the ever-present "experts" offering nonstandardized interventions such as testing of hair and urine for any of hundreds of potential toxins. Child health care providers may be presented with results of abnormal testing and a request to do something for the exposed child and family.

This article addresses air-quality science in the indoor environments in which children and adolescents find themselves, including the home, the school, and other environments such as work and recreational situations.

---

* Corresponding author.
E-mail address: manderso@dhha.org (M.E. Anderson).

0031-3955/07/$ - see front matter © 2007 Elsevier Inc. All rights reserved.
doi:10.1016/j.pcl.2007.01.003

pediatric.theclinics.com

Although the school arena is covered more extensively elsewhere in this issue of the *Pediatric Clinics of North America*, this article refers briefly to the importance of the school environment for children. The home arena is covered extensively, presenting an analysis of the usual exposures such as ETS and bioaerosols and also touching on discrete issues such as sudden infant death syndrome (SIDS), CO, and public housing. Other considerations such as recreation and work environments deserve attention and are covered as well.

The home arena

Environmental tobacco smoke

Decades of research incriminate smoking as a health hazard, and, more recently, environmental exposure to tobacco smoke also has been associated with a list of untoward health effects. A complete review of ETS as an important environmental issue for children cannot be presented appropriately in this brief section, but the relationship between ETS and asthma, SIDS, and other respiratory tract problems is discussed in more detail.

Although the consumption of tobacco products has declined consistently over the 4 decades since the first Surgeon General's report detailed the dangers associated with use of tobacco products, ETS remains an important indoor air issue for children. Consumption of tobacco products by adolescents and by certain minority populations, in particular, has been refractory to the declines in consumption witnessed by other demographic groups [1]. Public policy focusing on limiting advertising to vulnerable populations and on raising the price of tobacco products has met with some success, but approximately 20% to 25% of Americans continue to consume tobacco products regularly [1]. The home (and family car) environment may continue to provide a proximate dose of second-hand smoke [2], and many diseases and disease processes are worsened by this exposure.

Asthma is the most common chronic disease of children, and multiple environmental triggers cause or worsen asthma. National guidelines encourage the practitioner to identify and reduce or eliminate these environmental triggers in a comprehensive approach to pediatric asthma care [3]. ETS remains an important and potentially controllable risk factor for children who have asthma. The odds associating the presence of wheeze, cough, mucus production, and episodes of breathlessness with the diagnosis of asthma are greater in children of smokers [4]. Nocturnal asthma symptoms are increased [5], emergency department use is increased [6], asthma severity is worsened, lung function is decreased [7], and exacerbations are more frequent, in a dose–response manner [8], in asthmatic children who are exposed to ETS. Tobacco use and exposure is greatest among the lowest-income families, who also may experience barriers to accessing regular care. An already large but growing body of evidence incriminates smoking as a determinant of asthma morbidity, and any comprehensive intervention for asthma care must address this concern.

Many studies performed during the last 30 years have consistently identified a twofold increased odds of SIDS in association with maternal tobacco use during pregnancy [9–11]. Multiple independent risk factors have been identified also, including postnatal maternal and/or paternal smoking. A dose–response relationship exists, so that each cigarette smoked confers a 4% increased odds of SIDS to the newborn [12]. As prone sleeping, another major risk factor of SIDS, decreased in the 1990s, tobacco consumption by parents became the greatest risk factor for SIDS [12,13]. This exposure is preventable, and the pediatrician has an important role to assume in prevention of tobacco use [14,15].

Other diseases and disease processes in children are strongly influenced by ETS. Exposure to combustion products of tobacco increases the number of childhood ear infections and chronic middle ear effusions, increases the likelihood of lower respiratory tract infections such as bronchiolitis or pneumonia, increases illness duration, and can cause or contribute to chronic cough and persistent runny nose [4]. As an example of expensive, hospital-based expenditures related to ETS exposure, bronchiolitis occurs more commonly and more severely in children exposed to ETS. The EPA estimates that, for children younger than 18 months of age, an excess 150,000 to 300,000 hospitalizations for pneumonia or bronchitis occur annually in the United States because of ETS exposure [16].

What helps prevent exposure of children to ETS? Specifically, prevention works: never allow potential smokers to begin smoking. Work in California has demonstrated the unique economic vulnerability of adolescents as they initiate smoking. Although increasing the price of cigarettes results in decreased consumption for all age groups, consumption by adolescents decreases to a greater degree than that of adults in response to price-per-pack increases (www.tobaccofreealliane.org, [17,18]). Many, if not most, smokers begin smoking before age 20 years, and increased tobacco prices offer an obvious preventive measure to limit initiation.

Two additional interventions to protect children from ETS deserve mention. First, harm reduction is an often-practiced but poorly studied approach taken by pediatricians. This measure includes the reasonable advice to smoke outside and therefore never to smoke in the home or in the car where children may receive more concentrated exposure to ETS. Whether parents are capable of changing habits to engage in harm reduction practices and whether such practices result in demonstrable effects on children's disease processes is an area deserving inquiry. The advice to reduce harm seems quite reasonable, however. A second approach to limiting ETS exposure for children is to advise the adult smokers to quit smoking. Many pregnant mothers are able to quit smoking, but the recidivism rate is high [19,20]. The external pressure to quit smoking during pregnancy provides an excellent inducement. Quitting may be more difficult for other parents, who may have difficulty perceiving the link between their smoking and their child's illness. Pediatricians should use every opportunity to address ETS, ranging from the visit for a simple cold to an asthma exacerbation, to push parents toward considering the role their smoking has in the child's life. The pediatrician should understand what local resources are available, such as state-based programs created by the national tobacco settlement. These programs often include access to pharmaceuticals in addition to traditional counseling and support therapy used to encourage former smokers to remain tobacco free. The pediatrician has a key role in the quitting process: consider ETS as a component of the exposed child's problem list, and address it as a chronic illness.

Allergens and bioaerosols

Mold in the indoor environment receives much attention (see the article by Seltzer and colleagues in this issue). Separating fact from fiction is of utmost importance with mold, because many "solutions" are proposed to families to abate ubiquitous and naturally occurring molds. The EPA offers excellent guidance on mold in the home, including advice regarding appropriate do-it-yourself abatement and when to call a professional [21]. As with other aspects of the practice of pediatrics, prevention is key through quick control of water leaks and appropriate maintenance of home mechanical systems. Because mold requires water and food substrate to support growth, keeping water off the substrate prevents or limits mold growth. Several publications are available for additional information for health care providers [22,23].

Pets and pests may present a problem for sensitized children, such as children who have atopy or asthma. As with other exposures, abatement is the preferred approach, but many families may be unwilling to take this step. Pets with fur and dander should not be allowed into children's bedrooms, where children regularly spend more time than in any other location in the home. Among sensitized children in particular, reducing exposure to antigens such as dust mite and cockroach will reduce symptoms of asthma [24], and sensitized children are often multiply sensitized [25].

Chemicals in the indoor environment

Volatile organic chemicals (VOCs) are used widely in household products including paints and varnishes, cleaning and disinfecting agents, cosmetics, and fuels. The exposure can be limited or eliminated by buying only as much chemical as needed, following the manufacturer's guidelines, and appropriately discarding unused amounts of old chemicals. In particular, use of methylene chloride (in paint strippers, adhesive remover), benzene (in fuels, paint supplies, auto emissions, ETS), and perchloroethylene (from dry cleaning) should be limited [26]. This list certainly is not exhaustive, and use of any chemical indoors should be prudent and include measures to protect children from exposure.

Newly installed materials, such as carpet or furniture made of particleboard or pressed board, liberate chemicals for a period of time following manufacture and installation. The homeowner can discuss with the installer the options available to limit the associated odors (eg, rolling out the new product in a well-ventilated area before installation, use of low-emitting adhesives and low-VOC paints, and continued good ventilation of the affected area following installation). The concerned family might consider vacating the property for a short time.

Particulates

The combustion of hydrocarbons—natural gas, oil, wood, animal dung—for heating and cooking creates particulate pollution in the home. Wood and biomass fuels produce greater particulate loads but may be the only available heat source, particularly in the developing world. Exposure to particulate pollution in indoor air is associated with upper and lower airway disease and with other diseases such as disorders of the eye [27].

Industry has responded with devices designed to remove particulates for indoor air. Air purifiers in general function by one of two mechanisms: they either generate ozone and/or negative ions, or they filter the air pulled through the device. Ozone production in particular may serve to worsen ambient air rather than to purify it, and none of the tested machines was particularly effective at removing gas-phase pollutants (nitrogen dioxide, formaldehyde) in the indoor air. Ozone-generating "air purifiers" should not be used in homes, especially if someone has asthma. High-efficiency filters are effective at removing particulates from the air, but the filters require routine maintenance because efficiency decreases as the filter become clogged with the trapped particles [28].

Carbon monoxide

CO is truly a silent killer. An odorless gas created when hydrocarbons combust, CO continues to claim lives in the United States [29] and is responsible for more than 15,000 visits for medical care annually [30]. Worldwide, CO may explain up to one half of fatal poisonings, but the actual cases reflect underdetection and underreporting of the exposure. Symptoms are vague and nonspecific, but a high index of suspicion is life saving. Early symptoms of headache, dizziness, weakness, nausea, confusion, disorientation, and visual disturbances may be linked to a specific environment such as the home. Impaired oxygen transportation by carboxyhemoglobin results in hypoxia and its complications such as lethal arrhythmia. Delayed effects include impaired neuropsychiatric function beginning within days of the exposure and lasting for weeks [31]. The technology for detecting CO in the home environment has been available for many years, but use of such monitoring devices is neither ubiquitous nor universally mandated, although they are life saving.

Radon

Radon has become an indoor air-quality issue in the age of well-insulated housing. Radon is produced from the decay of uranium naturally present in the soil, is a heavier-than-air gas, and can accumulate in below-grade living areas where ventilation is poor. Inexpensive test kits are available (refer to EPA or state radon offices; eg, http://epa.gov/radon/), and abatement is possible but may involve some expense on the part of the homeowner. A spotlight shines on radon because of its link with lung cancer even with exposure in the home. Although the increased risk is small, radon exposure is so widespread that public health concern exists [32].

Housing as a mediator of physical health

A healthy child requires a healthy home. As a prototypical example, the disease course of asthma is influenced heavily by the home environment. Additional examples of harmful home exposures include lead, which can be a particularly important, but remediable, neurotoxin and other neurotoxicants, such as pesticides, which work by poisoning household pests and affect similar metabolic pathways in children. The quality of ventilation and the presence of mold, ETS, and pet dander in the home contribute to or detract from the health of a child. Exposure to multiple potentially harmful compounds may begin prenatally and continue through childhood, and any of these exposures may be more predominant in inner city homes, especially in public housing. Solutions for these exposures are readily available through abatement, discontinued use, or responsible and appropriate use. Knowledge gaps exist, in particular concerning the development of the complex nervous system of a child in the milieu of multiple exposures [33].

Other considerations

Children are special in many respects. For example, because of their greater relative metabolic demands that increase their need for water to drink and air to breathe and their unique interactions with the environment through hand-to-mouth behaviors, children deserve special surveillance and protection. Growth through childhood is not just physical growth but also involves the highly complex and programmed development of a central nervous system, the components of which communicate with each other by chemical signals. Lead exposure, even at low levels, provides an excellent example of how development is mildly but irreversibly interrupted in a vulnerable childhood window. Children are exposed to many manmade household chemicals that have unknown health profiles. Parents should be encouraged to help limit exposure by keeping chemicals out of the home.

Case presentation

A 12-year-old African American boy seeks care for an asthma attack. His moderate, persistent asthma has been well controlled for at least a couple of years, but he has experienced increasing exacerbations of asthma during the last 6 months. Two weeks earlier he was prescribed another course of prednisone for an asthma exacerbation. He presents again with increased wheezing and respiratory distress. He has been compliant on high-dose inhaled corticosteroid, intranasal steroids, and long-acting β-agonist and is using proper technique with his medications.

His family recently purchased and moved into their first home. The home, located in the inner city of a large metropolitan area, had been empty for a period of time after being used as a rental property. The patient's room was in the below-grade basement in the home. They had no pets, had seen no cockroaches, and denied use of tobacco products. When housing authorities visited the home, they found evidence of water damage caused by a leaking roof and mold growth in the kitchen and bathroom areas as well as in the basement. Fertilizer was stored in the basement and produced a strong chemical odor. The entire house was carpeted over hardwood flooring which, when pulled back, had large areas of burned hardwood. As the house's history unraveled, it had been used repeatedly while unoccupied for drug sales and use and had been fire bombed on one occasion. The then owner/landlord had cleaned the carpeting and painted the walls in preparation for sale.

Although this real case may sound extreme, it demonstrates the importance of the home environment as a determinant of health for children. Resources were identified to aid with home repair, interior cleaning, carpet removal, and refinishing of the hardwood floors. The child no longer sleeps in the basement of the house. Today the home no longer makes him sick, and his asthma has returned to baseline with good control. Many diseases are impacted by the indoor air quality surrounding children. The prudent pediatrician must remember to inquire about the environments in which children spend most or all of their time and take necessary steps to investigate these environments.

The school arena

Schools rank second on the list of indoor locations in which children spend the most time. Education is mandatory in the United States and for almost all children occurs in a setting outside the family home. As with housing in the United States, schools can be new or old, large or small, mobile or immobile. Creating and maintaining usable and safe structures in which to educate children and young adults is an ongoing challenge. Many schools are plagued by issues of ineffective indoor ventilation, problems with mold, lead, and asbestos, and the use of portable classrooms to meet issues of overcrowding and diminishing budgets. Many schools must function like miniature cities with needs for traffic control, safe food storage and preparation, and efficient waste disposal. Mixing these needs with the added entropy induced by children necessitates special attention to indoor air-quality issues in the schools.

Although this issue of the *Pediatric Clinics of North America* devotes an entire article to the discussion of schools and children's environmental health, schools deserve a brief mention here as part of a discussion of indoor air quality for children. Namely, what is known about the importance of school indoor air for children's health? If school is considered the occupation of childhood, how do these workers perform in their environment? In a 2002 review aiming to evaluate the quality and findings of research into the indoor school environment and its effects on children, the authors raised more questions than they answered. The available evidence suggested that indoor air quality has an influence on student performance, particularly in examination of indoor ventilation in the schools, but that further inquiry is needed [34]. Although the literature is still awaited, some resources are available now. The EPA and several partners have developed a schools-specific environmental quality workbook that includes considerations for indoor air quality, called the *Tools for Schools Action Kit* (http://www.epa.gov/IAQ/schools/tools). The workbook is intended for use as a comprehensive evaluation of a school's indoor environment ranging from food management to pest control. Childhood asthma receives special attention.

Other indoor environments

When evaluating children for potential sources of exposures, it is important to consider the different activities in which they engage and the particular environments in which they spend their time. Children may explore their surroundings, play or have hobbies, and some even work. The following sections highlight potential environmental sources to consider and their potential health impacts.

Children at play

The environments in which children develop have changed drastically in a single generation. Today children spend most of their time indoors (8- to 10-year-olds spend an average of 6 hours a day watching television, playing video games, and surfing the Internet [35]). This activity accounts for most of the time that children are not attending school or sleeping. Gone are the

days when children spent a large portion of their time playing outdoors do-
ing unstructured activities. Now outdoor time is limited and usually is reserved for specific activities such as sports on a set schedule. This
"internalization" of a child's play environment can lead to unique opportunities for exposures.

Homes contain a myriad of products, chemicals, and objects that offer
exposure hazards to children. The American Association of Poison Control
Centers reports that exposures to children aged less than 13 years account
for 58% of their annual human-exposure cases [36]. These exposures generally occur in the home and are mostly unintentional, acute, and result in
a minor effect. The five categories of substances most frequently involved
in pediatric exposures are cosmetics and personal care products, cleaning
substances, analgesics, foreign bodies, and topical agents. Measures should
be taken to safeguard against inadvertent exploration of kitchen and bathroom cabinets, closets, and garages where such products are usually stored.
A parent or health care provider can access the regional poison control center by a toll-free number (800-222-1222) to assist in evaluating an exposure
24 hours daily.

CO poisoning usually results from improper ventilation of certain
home heating devices but, along with elevated nitrogen dioxide, has
been also reported at indoor sporting venues including arenas for tractor
pulls, monster truck jumps, and ice rinks [37–39]. More than 300 persons,
mostly children, were exposed to CO (maximum detected levels reached
354 ppm) through exhaust fumes from a propane-powered ice-resurfacing
machine at an indoor rink [40]. Symptoms included fatigue, headache,
and dizziness, with 78 people requiring transport to a hospital. Carboxyhemoglobin levels ranged from 3.3% to 13.9%, and one 15-year-old with
symptoms of myocardial ischemia was referred for hyperbaric oxygen
therapy.

Tire crumb can be used indoors and outdoors to provide impact damp-
ening for playground surfaces. Because this material is derived from used
car tires, there has been concern about toxic metals and other components
leaching out of it. Toxicologic evaluations including hazard analyses, muta-
genicity assays, and aquatic toxicity tests indicate that there is minimal hazard for children from leachate or off-gassing [41].

Children at work

More than a third of high school–aged children work regularly during the
school year, and many more join the employed ranks during the summer
[42]. At age 12 years more than half of American youths reported some
type of work activity. For the period between 1996 and 1998 the Bureau
of Labor Statistics reported an average of 2.9 million workers aged 15 to
17 years worked during school months, and 4.0 million worked during summer months [43]. It is estimated that 200,000 workers annually between 14

and 17 years of age experience a job-related injury, requiring emergency treatment for 32% of these workers and resulting in 70 adolescent work-related deaths. Employment for these workers commonly includes restaurants, grocery stores, landscaping/gardening services, janitorial services, construction sites, and auto body/service stations [44].

Working as a lifeguard at an indoor pool may be the dream job of many adolescents, but it is not without potential risks. For example, the authors received a call from the parent of an 18-year-old male with a history of asthma who reported spells of weakness, chest pain, abdominal pain, and difficulty breathing. He worked at an indoor pool up to 40 hours per week and had to add the chlorine while wearing a mask. His symptoms improved away from work, and use of his albuterol inhaler provided no help with symptoms. Others working at the pool reported similar symptoms.

Research has indicated that inhaling levels of chlorine-based disinfectants as small as 0.02 to 0.20 ppm (as found around indoor pools) has been associated with increased prevalence of asthma after cumulative exposures, particularly in young children. Trichloramine can form when chlorine reacts with organic matter such as urine and sweat and may result in epithelial membrane damage such as increased blood concentrations of surfactant-associated proteins A and B [45]. Children spending increased time either swimming in or working at indoor pools may be at risk for inhalational exposures to chlorine compounds.

A common indoor work activity for youth across many industries is cleaning and use of cleaning products. Acute exposures to disinfectants and sanitizers usually involve inflammation, edema, and burns. The average incidence rate of acute occupational disinfectant-related illness for 15- to 17-year-olds from 1993 to 1998 was more than four times that of 25- to 44-year-olds. Illnesses were primarily mild-to-moderate in severity and did not differ between the two age groups. The use of personal protective gear was higher in adults than in youths [46].

Case reports of adolescent work-related fatalities and illness combined with observational studies of the increased risk of potential job-related chemical exposures suggest a need for better awareness of work-related exposures and illness among working youth. An additional need exists for better occupational safety training for working adolescents, education of parents and health care providers regarding these risks, clinical monitoring of all workers' health and safety, and advocacy for safer adolescent work environments [47–49].

Summary: improving the air quality in the home, at school, and at work

Pediatricians practice prevention-based medicine, recognizing that this is the most cost-efficient tool available and that health outcomes associated with prevention efforts are consistently better than those of secondary or tertiary prevention efforts. Indoor air quality is no exception: typically, the best way to improve indoor air quality is to eliminate the emission source. Home mechanical systems should be well maintained and used appropriately. Ventilation should be adequate to the home's requirements. Particulate-producing activities should be reduced or eliminated, or modifications to home ventilation and air cleaning may be necessary. Radon testing may be reasonable and can be done cheaply and quickly. Each home should have an appropriately placed and maintained CO detector. Tobacco smokers should quit or be encouraged to smoke only outside until they quit.

Pediatricians are challenged in many ways on a daily basis. The challenge with consideration of indoor air quality in acute or chronic illness is to picture the patient within an environmental milieu that may be causing or worsening an illness. Asthma is prototypical in this regard: asthma is truly an environmental disease, and any therapeutic approach to asthma must recognize the relevant environmental triggers and reduce or abate the exposures, or the child will not get better. Pediatricians should recognize that children's' environments are fluid as well, including the home environment and also occupational environments such as school and work place.

References

[1] Epidemiology Program Office, Office of the Director, CDC. Achievements in Public Health, 1900–1999: tobacco use—United States, 1900–1999. MMWR 1999;48(43):986–93.
[2] Reives D. Suffer the children. Chest 2002;122:394–6.
[3] US Department of Health and Human Services. NAEPP Expert Panel Report: guidelines for the diagnosis and management of asthma/update on selected topics, 2002. Bethesda (MD): Public Health Service; 2002.
[4] Johnston R, Burge H, Fisk W, et al. Committee on the Assessment of Asthma and Indoor Air, Division of Health Promotion and Disease Prevention, Institute of Medicine. Clearing the air: asthma and indoor exposures. Washington, DC: National Academy Press; 2002.
[5] Morkjaroenpong V, Rand C, Butz A, et al. Environmental tobacco smoke exposure and nocturnal symptoms among inner-city children with asthma. J Allergy Clin Immunol 2002;110: 147–53.
[6] Evans D, Levison M, Feldman C, et al. The impact of passive smoking on emergency room visits of urban children with asthma. Am Rev Respir Dis 1987;135:567–72.
[7] Mannino DM, Homa DM, Redd SC. Involuntary smoking and asthma severity in children. Chest 2002;122:409–15.
[8] Chilmonczyk B, Salmun L, Megathlin K, et al. Association between exposure to environmental tobacco smoke and exacerbations of asthma in children. N Engl J Med 1993; 328(23):1665–9.
[9] Comstock G, Shah F, Meyer M, et al. Low birth weight and neonatal mortality rate related to maternal smoking and socioeconomic status. Am J Obstet Gynecol 1971;111(1):53–9.
[10] Anderson HR, Cook DG. Passive smoking and sudden infant death syndrome: review of the epidemiological evidence. Thorax 1997;52:1003–9.
[11] Cnattingius S, Haglund B, Meirik O. Cigarette smoking as risk factor for late fetal and early neonatal death. Br Med J 1988;297:258–61.
[12] Anderson ME, Johnson DC, Batal HA. Sudden infant death syndrome and prenatal maternal smoking: rising attributed risk in the back to sleep era. BMC Med 2005;3:4.
[13] Kattwinkel J, Hauck F, Keenan M, et al. Task force on SIDS. The changing concept of SIDS: diagnostic coding shifts, controversies regarding the sleeping environment, and new variables to consider in reducing risk. Pediatrics 2005;116:1245–55.

[14] Kulig J, the Committee on Substance Abuse. Tobacco, alcohol, and other drugs: the role of the pediatrician in prevention, identification, and management of substance abuse. Pediatrics 2004;115:816–21.

[15] Committee on Substance Abuse. Tobacco's toll: implications for the pediatrician. Pediatrics 2001;107:794–8.

[16] Setting the record straight: secondhand smoke is a preventable health risk. US EPA publication #402-F-94-005. Washington, DC: Environmental Protection Agency; 1994.

[17] Chaloupka F. Pacula R. Changing adolescent smoking prevalence: the impact of price on youth tobacco use. Bethesda, MD: US Department of Health and Human Services, Public Health Service, National Institutes of Health, National Cancer Institute. Monograph # 14; November, 2001.

[18] Harris J, Connolly G, Brooks D, et al. Cigarette smoking before and after an excise tax increase and an anti-smoking campaign—Massachusetts, 1990–1996. MMWR 1996;45(44): 966–70.

[19] Orleans CT, Barker DC, Kaufman NJ. Helping pregnant smokers quit: meeting the challenge in the next decade. West J Med 2001;174:276–81.

[20] Lelong N, Kaminski M, Saurel-Cubiozolles M, et al. Postpartum return to smoking among usual smokers who quit during pregnancy. Eur J Public Health 2001;11(3):334–9.

[21] Mold remediation in schools and commercial buildings. EPA publication #402-K-01–001. Washington, DC: Environmental Protection Agency; 2001.

[22] Committee on Damp Indoor Spaces and Health. Damp indoor spaces and health. Washington, DC: The National Academies Press; 2004.

[23] Storey E, Dangman K, Schenck P, et al. Guidance for clinicians on the recognition and management of health effects related to mold exposure and moisture indoors. Farmington (CT): University of Connecticut Health Center; 2004.

[24] Morgan W, Crain E, Gruchalla R, et al. Result of a home-based environmental intervention among urban children with asthma. N Engl J Med 2004;351:1068–80.

[25] Crain E, Walter M, O'Connor G, et al. Home and allergic characteristic of children with asthma in seven US urban communities and design of an environmental intervention: the Inner City Asthma Study. Environ Health Perspect 2002;110(9):939–45.

[26] The inside story: a guide to indoor air quality. EPA publication #402-K-93–007. Washington, DC: Environmental Protection Agency; 1995.

[27] Ezzati M, Kammen D. Quantifying the effects of exposure to indoor air pollution from biomass combustion on acute respiratory infections in developing countries. Environ Health Perspect 2001;109:481–8.

[28] Manuel J. A healthy home environment? Environ Health Perspect 1999;107(7):A548.

[29] Office of Information and Public Affairs. NEWS from CPSC, release # 01–069. Washington, DC: US Consumer Product Safety Commission; 2001.

[30] Caravati E, Grey T, Nangle B, et al. Unintentional non-fire-related carbon monoxide exposures—United States, 2001–2003. MMWR 2005;54:36–9.

[31] Raub J, Mathieunolf M, Hampson N, et al. Carbon monoxide poisoning—a public health perspective. Toxicology 2000;145:1–14.

[32] Krewski D, Lubin J, Zielinski J, et al. Residential radon and risk of lung cancer: a combined analysis of 7 North American case-control studies. Epidemiology 2005;16(2):137–45.

[33] Breysse P, Farr N, Galke W, et al. The relationship between housing and health: children at risk. Environ Health Perspect 2004;112(15):1583–8.

[34] Heath G, Mendell M. Do indoor environments in schools influence student performance? A review of the literature. Proceedings: Indoor Air 2002;802–7.

[35] Cauchon D. Childhood pastimes are increasingly moving indoors. USA Today. July 12, 2005. Nation Section.

[36] Watson W, Litovitz T, Rodgers G, et al. Annual report of the American Association of Poison Control Centers Toxic Exposure Surveillance System. Am J Emerg Med 2004;22: 591–666.

[37] Smith W, Anderson T, Anderson H. Nitrogen dioxide and carbon monoxide intoxication in an indoor ice arena—Wisconsin. MMWR 1992;41:383–5.
[38] Boudreau D, Spadafora M, Wolf L, et al. Carbon monoxide levels during indoor sporting events—Cincinnati, 1992–1993. MMWR 1994;43:21–3.
[39] Lee K, Yanagisawa Y, Spengler J, et al. Carbon monoxide and nitrogen dioxide exposure in indoor skating rinks. J Sports Sci 1994;12:279–83.
[40] Hampson N. Carbon monoxide poisoning at an indoor ice risk and bingo hall—Seattle, 1996. MMWR 1996;45:265–7.
[41] Birkholz D, Belton K, Guidotti T. Toxicological evaluation for the hazard assessment of tire crumb for use in public playgrounds. J Air Waste Manag Assoc 2003;53:903–7.
[42] Rubenstein H, Sternbach M, Pollack S. Protecting the health and safety of working teenagers. Am Fam Physician 1999;60:575–87.
[43] Manser M, Kerschner A, Rothstein D, et al. Report on youth labor force. Washington, DC: US Department of Labor, Bureau of Labor Statistics; 2000.
[44] National Institute for Occupational Safety and Health. Request for assistance in preventing deaths and injuries of adolescent workers. DHHS Pub # 95–125. Cincinnati (OH): Department of Health and Human Services; 1995.
[45] Bernard A, Carbonnelle S, Michel O, et al. Lung hyperpermeability and asthma prevalence in school children: unexpected associations with attendance at indoor chlorinated swimming pools. Occup Environ Med 2003;60:385–94.
[46] Brevard T, Calvert G, Blondell J, et al. Acute occupational disinfectant-related illness among youth. Environ Health Perspect 2003;111:1654–9.
[47] Calvert G, Mehler L, Rosales R, et al. Acute pesticide-related illness among working youth. Am J Public Health 2003;93:605–10.
[48] Castillo D, Davis L, Wegman D. Young workers. Occup Med 1999;14:519–36.
[49] Pollack S. Adolescent occupational exposures and pediatric-adolescent take-home exposures. Pediatr Clin North Am 2001;48:1267–89.

ELSEVIER
SAUNDERS

Pediatr Clin N Am
54 (2007) 309–333

PEDIATRIC CLINICS
OF NORTH AMERICA

Health Effects of Mold in Children

James M. Seltzer, MD[a,b,*],
Marion J. Fedoruk, MD, CIH, DABT[a,c]

[a]Division of Occupational and Environmental Medicine, University of California, Irvine,
School of Medicine, 5201 California Avenue, Suite 100, Irvine, CA 92617 USA
[b]Pediatric Environmental Health Specialty Unit,
US Environmental Protection Agency Region IX, 5201 California Avenue,
Suite 100, Irvine, CA 92617, USA
[c]Center for Occupational & Environmental Health, Mail Code 1830,
5201 California Avenue, Suite 100, Irvine, CA 92617, USA

Fungi, ubiquitous unicellular or multicellular organisms of the Kingdom of Fungi, exist in several forms, including single-celled yeasts, microscopic filaments (hyphae), aggregates of these filaments (mycelia), and spore-producing visible fruiting bodies (eg, mushrooms). "Mold" and "mildew" are generic terms used to describe visible aggregates of hyphae that give fungi their fuzzy appearance. Fungi represent about 10% of the earth's biomass and serve to recycle organic matter. They grow on a wide variety of indoor and outdoor organic substrates, with water (moisture) the most important factor for determining growth for many species. Fungal components (FCs) include spores, hyphae, mycelia, allergenic sites (epitopes), and β-1,3-D-glucan, a principal component of the fungal cell wall. FCs can become airborne under ambient conditions, especially when mold is disturbed physically (eg, by air currents or mechanical disruption). Some molds have the ability to produce mycotoxins and are referred to as "toxigenic." Mycotoxins can be found in spores and hyphal fragments. Exposure to FCs occurs by inhalation, dermal contact, and ingestion. Mold growth indoors is very common. Respondents in a questionnaire study of white 9- to 11-year-olds in 24 communities across North America reported a prevalence of indoor mold growth of 22% to 57%, exceeding 50% of households in five communities [1].

As part of their professional activities, Drs. Seltzer and Fedoruk perform environmental and medical consulting. Some of this consulting involves forensic consulting, serving as a medical or environmental expert.

* Corresponding author. P.O. Box 1160, Oceanside, CA 92051.
  E-mail address: jseltzer@uci.edu (J.M. Seltzer).

Four types of pathogenic mechanisms have been linked to adverse health outcomes (AHOs) caused or exacerbated by molds: (1) immunologic reactions (2) toxicity, (3) infection, and (4) irritation. A fifth category, "indeterminate mechanism," might be added to account for AHOs, such as fatigue and headache, frequently associated with the presence of damp buildings or ambient mold for which the pathophysiologic mechanisms, if there indeed are any, remain undetermined.

The ability to define or exclude causal relationships between mold exposure and some AHOs is hindered by a number of factors too extensive to discuss in this article and more completely discussed in recent reviews [2–7]. The crux of the challenge is to define relevant FC exposure accurately and to measure the adverse health effects in humans designated for study while excluding confounding variables. Some factors interfering with the ability to elucidate relationships between mold and human morbidity are (1) inadequate knowledge about the health-relevant features of molds (eg, insufficient dose–response data), (2) the greater complexity of human sensitization and morbidity from molds relative to other harmful agents, (3) lack of a standardized methodology for assessing ambient FCs and some AHOs, and (4) inexact, inappropriate, or nonvalidated investigational methodology, (eg, use of nonvalidated self-report questionnaires). Furthermore, as a result of the recent prominence of mold in litigation as an alleged cause of illnesses ranging from asthma to autism, the ability of mold to cause human illness has received intense scrutiny. Despite these controversies and challenges, health care professionals continue to recognize mold as a cause or exacerbating factor in specific disorders and continue to evaluate and treat mold-induced illnesses using widely accepted clinical paradigms.

Adverse health outcomes—immunologic reactions

Three immunopathologic mechanisms have been identified as playing a role in the pathogenesis of hypersensitivity reactions caused by molds: (1) production of mold-specific serum IgE (immediate hypersensitivity), (2) antigen-specific antibody (IgG, IgM) forming immune complexes and activating inflammatory pathways in tissue, and (3) delayed hypersensitivity. A fourth mechanism, inflammation resulting from activation of the innate immune system by FCs, remains intriguing but as yet unproven in humans. Immediate hypersensitivity mechanisms are involved most frequently in the pathogenesis of asthma, rhinitis, eczema, and urticaria. In addition to the role of immediate hypersensitivity, nonimmunologic mechanisms (eg, viral infection and irritants in asthma) frequently contribute to AHOs for a given child who has one or more of these atopic diagnoses. Table 1 provides classical findings differentiating various hypersensitivity disorders. Deviation from these findings is common for many of these disorders.

The overall prevalence of fungal immunologic sensitization (the presence of specific IgE as opposed to atopic disease), ranging from 3% to 91% in the general population [8] and from 7% to 50% in children who have asthma [9–12], is complicated by varying study methodologies and the significant variability in the composition of mold extract allergens. In the general population of the United States the prevalence of *Alternaria* sensitization was reported to be 12.9% [13]. The antigenic epitopes of several molds, such as *Alternaria, Cladosporium, Aspergillus,* and *Penicillium,* have been characterized to varying degrees, and their role in the pathogenesis of allergic respiratory disease has been studied [14,15]. As with other allergens, mold sensitization develops in genetically predisposed individuals in response to recurrent or chronic environmental exposure [16]. Consistent with other classes of allergens, molds demonstrate cross-reactivity [8] (ie, the sharing of similar or identical antigenic sites [epitopes]) with other molds, for example, the enolases of *Cladosporium herbarum, Alternaria alternata, Saccharomyces cerevisiae, Candida albicans,* and *Aspergillus fumigatus* with some nonfungal allergens, such as latex.

Since the possibility was first proposed by Blackley [17] in 1873, scientists have suspected mold as one of several classes of inhaled allergens capable of causing or exacerbating asthma and other allergic respiratory disorders. The medical evaluation and treatment for mold-induced immediate hypersensitivity illnesses follows the methodology pursued for other allergens—a careful medical history to obtain symptom, exposure, and genetic information; a physical examination searching for signs of atopic disorders (eg, asthma, rhinitis, and eczema); skin or laboratory testing to determine allergic sensitization; and a treatment regimen consisting of reduced exposure, pharmacotherapy, and immunotherapy, when indicated. Cantani and Ciaschi [18], studying a population of 6840 atopic 1- to 9-year-old children living in Rome, Italy who had asthma and/or allergic rhinitis, found *A. alternata* sensitization in 3.3%, but monosensitization (no sensitization to the remainder of nonfungal allergens tested) in only 1.3% of the children. Based on the high prevalence of asthma in the 89 monosensitized children, the authors concluded *A. alternata* sensitization posed a significant independent risk factor for pediatric asthma. A prospective longitudinal study of nearly 1000 children in a semiarid climate found *A. alternata* sensitization at age 6 years was the only allergen independently associated with an increased risk of asthma at both age 6 years (odds ratio = 2.3) and 11 years (odds ratio = 2.7) [10]. In a large, multicenter, cross-sectional study of 1041 children who had mild-to-moderate asthma, 88% demonstrated at least one positive skin prick test (SPT) to a panel of inhalant allergens, including 37% to *A alternata*, 24% to *Penicillium* mix, and 22% to *Aspergillus* mix. The authors found the strongest associations of increased bronchial hyperreactivity (PC_{20} with methacholine challenge) with allergic sensitization to dog ($P = .003$), *Alternaria* ($P = .01$), and cat ($P = .05$). The investigators concluded that their findings support the important role sensitization to these allergens plays in modulating bronchial responsiveness [19]. A number of other reports have found sensitization to *Alternaria* to be a significant independent risk factor

Table 1
Mold-induced hypersensitivity disorders: comparison of findings

Condition	Asthma	Total IgE	Mold-specific IgE	Specific IgG	Peripheral eosinophilia	Lung Function	Imaging	Other findings
Allergic rhinitis	+ or –	↑ or wnl	↑	Irrelevant	+ or –	wnl		
Allergic asthma	+	↑ or wnl	↑	Irrelevant	+ or –	Normal or large or small airway obstruction	Chest radiograph: hyperaeration or wnl	
Nonatopic asthma	+	↑ or wnl	–	Irrelevant	+ or –	Normal or large or small airway obstruction	Chest radiograph: hyperaeration or wnl	
Acute allergic bronchopulmonary mycosis/allergic bronchopulmonary aspergillosis	+	↑↑(> 1000 IU/mL)	↑	Precipitins	+	1. Airway obstruction 2. Restrictive defect (if lung fibrosis)	Chest radiograph: infiltrates Chest CT: usually central bronchiectasis	Aspergillus hyphae in sputum
Allergic fungal sinusitis		Usually ↑–↑↑	+ by skin testing – in serum	↑ but no serum precipitins	–	wnl	Sinus CT: 1. Mucosal hypertrophy 2. Hyperattenuation of sinus contents often present 3. In children: more often unilateral and asymmetric, and bony abnormalities	1. Extramucosal allergic mucin 2. Scattered fungal hyphae or fungal culture + 3. Eosinophilic-lymphocytic sinus mucosal inflammation 4. No tissue invasion 5. Nasal polyps

HEALTH EFFECTS OF MOLD IN CHILDREN   313

Hypersensitivity pneumonitis	—	wnl	—	Precipitins, often multiple. Infrequently —	—	1. Restrictive defect 2. Airway obstruction (sometimes) 3. ↓ DLCO	Chest radiograph: diffuse micronodular infiltrates Chest high-resolution CT: 1. Ground-glass opacities and/or centrilobular nodules 2. Fibrosis (later stage)	BAL: Lymphocytosis Histopathology: Smaller non-caseating granulomas, loosely arranged and less well defined, peri-alveolar

Abbreviations: BAL: bronchoalveolar lavage; DLCO, diffusing capacity of lung for carbon monoxide; wnl, within normal limits; −, negative; +, positive; ↑, elevated; ↓, decreased.

for the development or persistence of asthma in children [14,20,21] and for respiratory arrest in asthmatic children and young adults [22]. In a prospective study in Norway, Nilsson and Aas [23] identified 53 atopic asthmatic children age 6 to 15 years with positive bronchoprovocation tests to mold extracts of *C. herbarum*. In this study SPTs predicted allergic asthma from *Cladosporium* sensitivity in 83% to 96% of cases compared with 74% to 83% for the radioallergosorbent assay test. Similar increased adverse health effects on asthma in adults have been described for indoor mold growth [24].

Although antigen-specific immunotherapy has been used to treat mold allergy for years, only a few studies have evaluated its efficacy. Desensitization with standardized *Cladosporium* extracts in polysensitized adults and children has been shown to reduce bronchial or conjunctival challenge reactivity in *Cladosporium*-sensitive asthma or rhinoconjunctivitis, but demonstration of improvement in symptom-medication scores was questionable [25–27]. In a double-blind, placebo-controlled immunotherapy study with 20 adult and pediatric patients having allergic rhinitis (42% of whom also had asthma) monosensitized to *Alternaria*, Horst and colleagues were able to show statistically significant improvement in several parameters following active treatment: patient self-assessment of efficacy, global symptom-medication scores, rhinitis scores, reduced skin test and nasal challenge reactivity [28]. The authors noted the difficulty in finding monosensitized patients to evaluate. Additional studies of desensitization in *Alternaria*-sensitive respiratory tract disease have shown benefit [29,30].

Studies of documented mold-sensitive asthmatics provide evidence-based support for the role of mold sensitivity in allergic disease of the upper airways and conjunctiva, because many children who have asthma have concomitant allergic rhinoconjunctivitis [14,18,28]. Few studies have targeted children who have allergic rhinoconjunctivitis and mold sensitivity. Nineteen percent of 202 children ages 2 to 14 years who had allergic rhinitis living in a tropical environment were SPT positive to one or more molds in a standard testing battery of various types of inhalant allergens. Mold sensitization was significantly more prevalent in houses without air conditioning (odds ratio = 9.4) and usually presented with polysensitization to three or more molds [31]. *Alternaria* sensitivity was associated with increased amounts of leukotriene C4 (LTC4), an inflammatory mediator of phospholipids metabolism, in the nasopharyngeal secretions of children with ragweed sensitivity during the ragweed pollen season. Increased levels of LTC4 continued after the end of the ragweed season, coincident with peaks of mold spore counts [32], supporting a role for mold exposure in allergic inflammation. Stark and colleagues [33] reported infants with a positive family history for atopy exposed to high levels of dust-borne fungi are at increased risk of developing allergic rhinitis by 5 years of age. Mold sensitivity also may be an important risk factor for the development of adenoidal hypertrophy [34] or sinusitis [35] in children who have allergic rhinitis. If not well controlled, the discomfort, frustration, and fatigue that may be caused by symptoms from allergic hypersensitivity disorders from any allergen, including mold, can result in cognitive impairment (eg, decreased vigilance, slowed mental processing) and reduced quality of life by interfering with sleep (sedation), causing distraction, and inducing or aggravating mood disorders [36–39].

Scientific validation of the role of molds in the pathophysiology of atopic dermatitis (atopic eczema) and urticaria is sparse. In one study, 15 of 30 children who had atopic dermatitis (AD) but only 2 of 30 children who had respiratory allergy but no AD developed eczematous lesions upon patch testing with a mold mix [40]. Clark and Adinoff [41] found patients who had AD, but not controls who had allergic rhinitis, demonstrated patch test–positive delayed cutaneous reactions to various inhalant allergens, including molds, for which they were SPT positive. They concluded aeroallergen contact plays an important role in select patients who have AD. Sampson [42], reviewing the role of allergy in AD, cautioned that, although a few studies provide strong evidence for an etiologic role for mold in AD, further studies are needed to evaluate clinical significance. Two case reports have suggested inhalation or ingestion of *Aspergillus* [43] or *Boletus edulis* (an edible basidiomycete) [44] to which subjects were sensitized resulted in IgE-mediated anaphylactic reactions. Maibach [45] reported the development of contact urticaria from mold exposure.

Allergic bronchopulmonary mycosis (ABPM) is a pulmonary disorder caused by IgE- and immune complex–mediated mold hypersensitivity characterized by asthma, fleeting pulmonary infiltrates, pulmonary and peripheral blood eosinophilia, saprophytic fungal growth in the lower airways without invasion, and a good clinical response to systemic corticosteroids [46–48]. High-resolution CT scans of the chest usually identify central (proximal) bronchiectasis in later stages of the disease. Patients who have ABPM are immunocompetent and almost uniformly demonstrate highly elevated total serum IgE (usually >600 IU/ml), increased amounts of mold-specific IgE by skin testing or in vitro testing, and mold-specific IgG precipitins in serum and/or lung. Allergic bronchopulmonary aspergillosis is the predominant form of ABPM. Allergic bronchopulmonary aspergillosis (ABPA), however, represents only a small subset of *A. fumigatus*–sensitive patients who have asthma (1%–2%) or cystic fibrosis (7%–9%) [49–51]. ABPA is not rare in children and has even been reported in infants [46,52]. All of the classical criteria may be absent in some patients who have ABPM [46]. Pediatric cases of ABPM attributable to other fungi have been described for *Bipolaris, C. albicans, Curvularia, Pseudoallescheria boydii*, and *Fusarium vasinfectum* [53,54]. Treatment consists of allergen avoidance, treatment of asthma, and courses of oral corticosteroids for refractory lung disease.

Allergic fungal sinusitis shares several histopathologic, laboratory, and clinical features with ABPM. First described by Katzenstein and colleagues [55], allergic fungal sinusitis presents with hypertrophic unilateral or bilateral chronic sinusitis that usually is resistant to treatment with antihistamine/decongestants, antibiotics, and topical anti-inflammatory agents. Classic features include nasal obstruction, nasal polyps, saprophytic fungal growth without tissue invasion, and thick, eosinophil-laden, peanut butter–like sinus masses and nasal casts of allergic mucin. Accumulation of the allergic mucin sometimes results in destruction of bony elements by mass expansion into the orbit or cranial fossae in the absence of fungal tissue invasion. The allergic mucin has a characteristic heterogeneous or attenuating appearance as sinus opacification on CT scanning, and the sinus contents demonstrate positive fungal staining or culture. As in ABPM, total serum IgE often is quite high with demonstrable levels of specific IgE by skin testing but less frequently in serum. Usually, specific IgG for the offending mold is present, although precipitins usually are absent [56–60]. More commonly than in adults, children who have allergic fungal sinusitis are male (ratio of 2.1 versus 0.7 in adults), present with facial dysmorphism (42% versus 10%), unilateral disease (70% versus 37%), asymmetrical disease (88% versus 58%), and sensitivity to fungi other than *Aspergillus* (0% versus 13%) [61]. *Bipolaris* species has been most commonly identified, particularly in the Southwest and inland parts of the United States, with *Curvularia* predominating in the Southeast [57]. *Aspergillus* was the only mold identified in a series from India [62]. Treatment usually consists of endoscopic evacuation of sinus contents with débridement of the affected tissue, may include irrigation with an antifungal antibiotic in saline, and, postoperatively, close follow-up, further débridement as needed, topical and judicious use of oral corticosteroids for an extended period of time, and treatment of underlying allergic disease [59,63].

Hypersensitivity pneumonitis (HP), also termed "extrinsic allergic alveolitis," is an uncommon but underdiagnosed disorder characterized by (1) exposure to organic dust antigens or certain low molecular weight chemical compounds, (2) a characteristic clinical presentation including abnormalities in lung function and imaging, and (3) laboratory evidence of immune complex and delayed-type hypersensitivity [64]. Children can present with the acute onset of fever, dry cough, malaise, chills, and dyspnea after antigen exposure (acute form). These symptoms generally resolve over 12 to 48 hours after removal from the offending antigen. The chronic form usually is characterized by a slow insidious progression of dyspnea, weight loss, fever, and cough over a period of years. Subacute and subacute chronic forms exist with some characteristics of both acute and chronic forms of the disease [65]. Physical examination may be normal, but often bibasilar crackles are heard over the lung fields, and clubbing may be present with the chronic form. Pulmonary function testing usually demonstrates a restrictive deficit, sometimes with an airway obstruction component. Diffusing capacity is reduced, often with resulting hypoxemia, especially with exercise. Abnormalities in dynamic lung compliance and diffusing capacity can persist for months following removal from the offending antigen(s) [66]. Pulmonary hypertension may develop with longstanding disease, but in children can reverse completely with successful treatment. Radiographic findings may be absent or show fleeting fine, reticular infiltrates or evidence of end-stage fibrosis. High-resolution CT scan of the chest provides the most accurate diagnostic radiographic assessment, showing micronodules predominantly in the upper and middle lung field and widespread ground-glass appearance. Laboratory findings in adults usually include the presence of precipitating IgG antibody (precipitins) against one or more antigens detectable by agar double-diffusion assay and T-lymphocytosis with decreased CD4+/CD8+ ratio in bronchoalveolar lavage (BAL) fluid. Lung biopsy demonstrates predominantly mononuclear cell infiltration of small airways and pulmonary parenchyma, often with poorly formed granulomas. Although precipitins can be found in as many as 50% of individuals exposed to high levels of the antigen, only a small proportion with this finding (eg, 5% in pigeon breeders) develops disease [67]. Conversely, precipitins were found in only 89% of children who had the diagnosis of HP [64]. Ratjen and colleagues [68] reported finding lymphocytosis with normal CD4+/CD8+ ratios in BAL fluid in nine children aged 6 to 15 years old who had HP; molds were the inciting antigens in four of these children. Failure to make the diagnosis and to eliminate exposure to the offending antigen(s) often results in progression to end-stage interstitial and intra-alveolar fibrosis. The predominant allergens causing HP have been avian proteins, particularly from pigeons, but fungi (eg, *Aspergillus* [66,68–70], *Penicillium, Alternaria, Cryptostroma, Pullularia, Rhodotorula* [65], *Cladosporium* [71], *Epicoccum* [72], *Fusarium* [73], and *Trichosporon cutaneum* [74,75]) have been associated with development of this disorder.

Hypersensitivity disorders are created by dysfunction of adaptive immunity, that is, antigen-specific immune responses. Another arm of the immune system, innate immunity, responds nonspecifically to pathogen-associated molecular patterns common to a range of external threats (eg, β-1,3-D-glucan). These foreign pathology-associated molecular patterns (PAMPs) can induce immediate inflammatory responses from the innate immune system and also can activate mechanisms of adaptive immunity downstream [76–78]. β-1,3-D-glucan, a polyglucose structural component in the cell walls of molds, can affect mononuclear cell cytokine production and induce inflammation in mice and guinea pigs [79–82]. Holt [82] hypothesized that the binding of β-1,3-D-glucan to receptors on antigen-presenting cells, such as monocytes and dendritic cells, could modulate cytokine production by these cells and skew T-lymphocyte function toward a T-helper cell type 2 (atopic) predominance. Evaluations of changes in secretion of inflammatory mediators by peripheral blood monocytes after β-1,3-D-glucan inhalation in healthy individuals and people living in damp buildings with high or low levels of airborne β-1,3-D-glucan have demonstrated variable and inconsistent responses [83–85]. Hirvonen and colleagues [86] found bacterial strains from moldy buildings were more potent inducers of inflammation than molds, although

Fogelmark and colleagues [81] found equivalent responses to inhaled solubilized β-1,3-D-glucan in guinea pigs. A recent review of the scientific evidence concluded that the data suggest some association between β-1,3-D-glucan exposure, airway inflammation, and symptoms [87], but larger observational studies using validated environmental assessment assays for β-1,3-D-glucan exposure are necessary to determine the nature and strength of any association. Fungal allergens from molds such as *Aspergillus* and *Alternaria* contain proteases with inflammatory modulatory effects in animals and in vitro [88,89], but their relevance to human disease remains unclear. Other fungi-associated molecular patterns with potential relevance to human inflammation and disease include several mannoproteins and zymosan [76,77].

Adverse health effects—toxicity

Mycotoxins are fungal intermediary metabolic products secreted extracellularly to provide a competitive growth advantage against other microbes. Higher organisms, including humans, can develop toxicity from some of these compounds. There are hundreds of mycotoxins with diverse chemical structures that can be produced by different fungal species. Genetic and environmental factors affecting synthesis include moisture, temperature, substrate, presence of competing organisms, and growth cycle. Mycotoxin production varies within species: not all strains of fungal species produce mycotoxins. Fungi having the potential to produce mycotoxins are assigned the label "toxigenic."

Mycotoxin exposure is ubiquitous in human populations. Mycotoxins are regularly found in grains, cereals, nuts, and animal products, including meat, eggs, and milk. Mycotoxins found in foods include trichothecenes, fumonisins, ochratoxin A, aflatoxins, and zearalones. Mycotoxins have produced human disease for centuries. The term "mycotoxicosis" refers to a disease caused by mycotoxin exposure. Examples of food-borne outbreaks include alimentary toxic aleukia and ergotism from ingestion of bread made of rye infested with *Claviceps purpura*. Alimentary toxic aleukia is a radiation-like illness that developed in the 1930s from ingestion of T2 mycotoxin elaborated by *Fusarium* in over-wintered grain among impoverished Eastern Europeans. Food-related mycotoxin illnesses occur primarily in Third World countries. Mycotoxins found in toxic mushrooms can produce serious illness and death, and children may inadvertently ingest them. Mushroom mycotoxins of clinical concern include cyclopeptides, orellanine, muscarine, hallucinogenic indoles, monomethylhydrazine, and isoxazoles.

There has been considerable controversy concerning whether mycotoxins from building exposures produce disease [6]. Some of this controversy can be attributed to the dearth of currently available data addressing the issue of causation and the difficulties with methodology. Fungi associated with damp buildings having the potential to produce mycotoxins include certain *Penicillium* and *Aspergillus* species, *Stachybotrys chartarum*, *Trichoderma*, and *Chaetomium* species. Toxic health outcomes attributed to building-related exposures include respiratory, immune, and neurologic effects [90,91]. The evidence for building-related mycotoxic illness, however, is limited to anecdotal case reports or limited epidemiologic studies that have many deficiencies [4,92]. Although a few publications have attributed human disease to inhalation or absorption (through skin) of mycotoxins [93], reviews of the medical literature concerning building-associated mycotoxic illness generally reveal an overall consensus that, at this time, credible scientific evidence for non–food-borne mycotoxin-induced human disease is lacking [6,7,92,94–97]. Other factors supporting the lack of effect include the limited doses that can be received by persons from a building-related exposure [98]. Furthermore, mycotoxins that contaminate animal feeds or are produced in laboratory settings are rarely, if ever, found in indoor environments [99].

Building-associated mycotoxin exposure was reported to be the cause of an outbreak of acute idiopathic pulmonary hemorrhage in African American infants. Cases initially were attributed to mycotoxin exposure from growth of *S. chartarum* in water-damaged homes in Cleveland, Ohio [100,101]. In a reassessment of the original study findings, however, the Centers for Disease Control identified several shortcomings in the methodology and the data interpretation employed to reach the initial causal conclusion. Consequently, the Centers for Disease Control retracted its initial conclusion, stating the association between acute idiopathic pulmonary hemorrhage and *S. chartarum* was not proven. The cause or causes of this unusual cluster remains undetermined. Despite a lack of reasonable scientific evidence to support *Stachybotrys*-induced human disease, proponents continue to cite anecdotal evidence as proof of a likely causal link, especially for pulmonary hemorrhage in infants [102–104]. Subsequent animal studies investigating the pulmonary toxicity effects [105,106] of *Stachybotrys* spores suffer from a number of limitations, making analogy with potential human illness tenuous [92,107].

A practical methodology to assess environmental levels of mycotoxins is needed. Environmental test results measuring mycotoxin in materials found in bulk samples collected from buildings correlate poorly with exposure [108]. Methodologies to measure human exposure, such as antibody tests to measure mycotoxin-specific antibody levels of various immunoglobulin classes in serum, have not been validated and are not indicated for clinical use [108,109]. Studies involving measurement of mycotoxins in blood and urine are being assessed to evaluate potential mycotoxin exposure and dose [110,111]. Development of biologic assays for mycotoxins in humans and environmental media that are indicative of exposure potential are key factors in understanding better the relationships between mycotoxic effects and environmental exposures. The complex process of describing the events from environmental contaminant source, including mycotoxins, to human response is illustrated in Table 2.

"Organic dust toxic syndrome" is a term used to describe an acute febrile illness characterized by flulike symptoms including chills, malaise, myalgia,

Table 2
A generalization of the aerobiologic pathway leading to inhalation exposure

Source factors →	Aerosol factors →	Exposure factors →	Response factors
The organisms	Composition of	Time spent in	Dose reaching
Populations, their	aerosols	aerosol	appropriate
interactions and	Particle size	Breathing rate	organ
dynamics	distribution	Particle deposition	Dose needed
Chemistry, physiology,	Dispersion	sites	for effect
biology of the	Biologic decay	Clearance rates	Metabolism of
organisms	Physical decay	Metabolic	toxin
Particle release factors	Patterns of aerosol	destruction	Human
	concentration	of toxin	susceptibility
			factors

From Burge HA. Fungi: toxic killers or unavoidable nuisances? Ann Allergy Asthma Immunol 2001;87(6 Suppl 3):52–6; with permission.

cough, and dyspnea following large exposures to organic dusts contaminated with micro-organisms, including molds and bacteria [112]. Pneumonia does not occur, and the condition resolves without sequelae. It occurs primarily following large organic dust exposures, especially moldy grain, hay, straw, and wood chips [113]. One report related exposure to dense airborne dust from a hay-covered floor at a college party resulted in the development of organic dust toxic syndrome [114]. A high attack rate is observed in persons with heavy exposure. Sensitization to an antigen is not required. Several causal agents have been implicated including endotoxin and β-1,3-D-glucan. Although organic dust toxic syndrome generally occurs in occupational agricultural settings where sufficiently large amounts of organic dust are present, this diagnosis should be considered in individuals experiencing these symptoms in highly contaminated indoor environments [6].

Adverse health effects—infection

Extensive reviews of fungal infections are available in the literature and are not covered in the print version of this article [108,115–121].

Adverse health effects—irritation

The fourth mechanism of mold-induced injury, irritation, has been less well studied than the first three. The olfactory (CN I), trigeminal (CN V), glossopharyngeal (CN IX), and vagal (CN X) nerves provide sensory afferents to the upper respiratory tract. C- and Aδ-nociceptive fibers make up the terminal branches of the trigeminal nerve endings in conjunctival and airway mucosa [122–125]. Volatile organic compounds (VOCs; MVOCs when from microbial sources) have been identified as possible causes of some of the AHOs attributed to mold exposure, presumably mediated through these irritant receptors. The evidence implicating MVOCs is sparse, however. Nilsson and colleagues [126] identified VOCs known to be produced by the molds *Aspergillus, Penicillium,* and *Cladosporium* adsorbed to airborne dust particles in both dry and damp residences. None of the occupants had health complaints, however, and no differences were noted between damp and dry residences in VOCs or mold spore concentrations per gram of dust. Another study investigating the role of home dampness and VOC concentrations on occupants' sick building syndrome (SBS) symptoms [127] found significantly increased odds ratios for the presence of dampness, several individual VOCs, and total VOCs for various types of symptoms referable to skin, eyes, the upper respiratory tract, and general symptoms (eg, fatigue, headache, dizziness). Problems with the study design included assessment of both building dampness and symptoms by questionnaire completed by occupants, which potentially would bias toward the positive any relationship between dampness and symptoms. Additionally, as the authors point out, the levels of VOCs they found were relatively low. There are other confounding factors in the evaluation of VOCs:

1. The conditions that promote mold growth (ie, excessive moisture and organic nutrient sources) promote the growth of other micro-organisms, such as bacteria and dust mites, each having its own potential for producing AHOs.
2. Dampness and VOCs produced by water-damaged building materials also may contribute to the development of AHOs.

Future studies of AHOs in larger groups of subjects with measurable exposure to MVOCs of fungal origin and careful characterization of the fungal flora of the contaminated space will be required to establish any causal relationships for MVOCs

Possible adverse health effects—indeterminate mechanisms

SBS consists of a constellation of mainly subjective health complaints such as headache, mucous membrane irritation, cognitive complaints (eg, memory loss, difficulty concentrating), and fatigue attributed to factors in a building that cannot be related to an established, scientifically valid diagnosis [128]. SBS has been described most commonly in adult office workers; reports of SBS affecting children are rare. Mold is one of a number of agents or conditions suggested as a possible cause of SBS, including cognitive impairment. Reports of mold exposure associated with complaints of SBS [129–131] and cognitive impairment [132] have been deficient in a number of areas (eg, failing to provide details of the prevalence and nature of health complaints, poor characterization of mold exposure, and failure to consider or investigate other possible causes of AHOs such as endotoxin [especially at zoological sites], dust mites, and VOCs). Psychogenic factors may contribute to the pathogenesis or exacerbation of AHOs in mold-contaminated buildings [133–135]. No scientifically sound data support a role for mold in the pathogenesis of SBS, the causes for which remain elusive and probably are multifactorial.

Dampness in buildings facilitates mold growth but also facilitates the growth of other microbial agents with AHO potential, such as bacteria and dust mites. Moisture can degrade building materials and furnishings, releasing VOCs with the potential to cause irritant responses and, if excessive, can cause physical discomfort. Criteria used to deem a residence damp or moldy vary among studies. The reported prevalence of "damp or moldy" dwellings in studies has ranged from 14.1% to 64%, and the reported prevalence of "mold growth" has ranged from 20% to 57% [1,136–139]. Numerous reports have found associations between dampness and/or mold and AHOs. Some of these reports have attempted to differentiate the effects of dampness from other possible dampness-related causes, such as mold and dust mite (Box 1) [6].

Methodologic and technological problems, too extensive for this article and discussed elsewhere in the literature, sometimes have hindered reliable accurate measurement of the responsivity of building occupants or the adequate characterization of exposure levels to mold and fungal components in the environment. These difficulties have, to varying degrees, confounded the determination of causal relationships [2,4–7,140]. Investigators often have not identified offending agents or explained the pathogenic mechanism(s) for conditions demonstrating statistically significant associations with AHOs (eg, dampness and lower respiratory tract symptoms). Despite these obstacles, it seems that dampness and/or mold exposure in some, as yet, undefined manner can exacerbate or might cause AHOs such as cough, phlegm, wheeze, dyspnea, pneumonia, bronchitis, sore throat, asthma, allergic rhinitis, and acute otitis media. Odds ratios for the risk of the development of upper or lower respiratory tract complaints (doctor diagnosed or self reported) associated with dampness and/or mold exposure range greatly, from insignificant to highly statistically significant, depending on the outcomes measured and the study design [6,127,136,141–147]. Peat and colleagues [146], in a review of the literature, reported an odds ratio ranging from 1.5 to 3.5 for wheeze or chronic cough in children living in damp or moldy homes, with larger sample sizes more likely to be statistically significant. In a study of 165 children 7 to 8 years of age in Edinburgh, Scotland, Strachan and Elton [144] discovered statistically significant associations for nocturnal cough, wheezing, family history of wheezing, and school absence from chest problems with mold and/or dampness in the home. They also remarked about possible reporting bias in the records of the children's general practitioners, in which this highly significant relationship was not found. Spengler and colleagues [1] concluded it was "highly probable" the presence of mold and damp conditions in homes contributed to the statistically significant increase in lower respiratory tract symptoms in their study population from a questionnaire-based study of white children 9

Box 1. Summary of findings regarding the association between health outcomes and exposure to damp indoor environments[1]

Sufficient evidence of a causal relationship
No outcomes met this definition

Sufficient evidence of an association
Upper respiratory tract (nasal and throat) symptoms
Cough
Whceze
Asthma symptoms in sensitized asthmatic persons

Limited or suggestive evidence of an association
Dyspnea (shortness of breath)
Lower respiratory illness in otherwise healthy children
Asthma development

Inadequate or insufficient evidence to determine whether an association exists
Airflow obstruction (in otherwise-healthy persons)
Mucous membrane irritation syndrome
Chronic obstructive pulmonary disease
Inhalation fevers (nonoccupational exposures)
Lower respiratory illness in otherwise-healthy adults
Acute idiopathic pulmonary hemorrhage in infants
Skin symptoms
Gastrointestinal tract problems
Fatigue
Neuropsychiatric symptoms
Cancer
Reproductive effects
Rheumatologic and other immune diseases

---

[1] These conclusions are not applicable to immunocompromised persons, who are at increased risk for fungal colonization or opportunistic infections.

Data from The Institute of Medicine of the National Academies. Damp indoor spaces and health. Washington, DC: The National Academies Press; 2004.

---

to 11 years of age in 24 communities across North America. They cautioned about the importance of reducing the risk of responder bias in this type of study by comparing self-reported symptoms with a set of objective measures. Some of these studies have also found associations between dampness or mold and various nonrespiratory symptoms such as fatigue, headache, nausea, dizziness, fever, and difficulty concentrating [127,136]. Some of these studies have reported dose–response relationships between damp/mold exposure and AHOs [136,147]. Objective measurements of lung function, however, have not correlated well with the presence of dampness or mold [138,148]. Bornehag and colleagues [149] reported that their evaluation of 61 epidemiologic peer-reviewed articles supported (1) a causal association between indoor "dampness" and lower respiratory tract symptoms (eg, cough, wheeze, and asthma), and (2) a more tenuous association between dampness and general symptoms (eg, fatigue, headache) despite an undetermined pathogenesis. The Institute of Medicine's [6] most recent report arrived at the conclusion of an "associational" but not "causal" relationship between dampness and both lower and upper respiratory tract symptoms (Box 1).

Damp or mold-contaminated conditions at schools present a potentially significant public health problem for children and employees [150]. Children at such schools generally are not free simply to pick up and move to another school; they must remain in the school environment. Excessive moisture or mold growth in schools has been associated with a statistically significant increased risk of asthma, upper and lower respiratory tract symptoms, and infections [9,151–154]. Atopy to inhalant allergens other than molds may be an additional risk factor for increased coughing in children in mold-contaminated schools [151]. Conversely, mold exposure in elementary schools has been suggested as a possible factor in increasing IgE sensitization to non-fungal inhalant allergens as well as the development of newly reported allergic disease [155]. Other building-related symptoms (ie, eye and throat irritation, headache, and dizziness) have been significantly associated with total viable mold concentrations in floor dust from schools in adolescent children [156], but not in postmenarchal girls [157]. Scheel and colleagues [158] attributed the presence of "SBS symptoms" in students and staff to *Stachybotrys* growth at a school with indoor water damage. Description of specific symptoms, characterization of exposure, and response to removal from exposure were lacking, however. Adding to the complexity of determining valid causal relationships is the need for scientific investigation to consider the potential for seasonal variations in the concentrations and proportional representation of mold genera [159]. This factor can affect indoor and outdoor mold concentrations in schools in the absence of evidence of visible mold growth or excessive moisture. To assist with identifying and correcting these problems, the Environmental Protection Agency has published "Mold Remediation in Schools and Commercial Buildings," available at http://www.epa.gov/mold/mold_remediation.html.

Summary

Mold is ubiquitous. Children are exposed to mold spores and other FCs every day, whether they are outdoors or indoors. Consequently, depending on a child's genotype and underlying health status, mold exposure, regardless of source, has the potential to produce AHOs. Certain states of health, notably pre-existing hypersensitivity and immunosuppression, place the child at increased risk of developing illness as a result of mold exposure. The four types of mechanisms by which molds can produce human illness are immunologic reactions, toxicity, infection, and irritation. Several recent reviews of the literature have concluded insufficient valid scientific data exist to establish epidemiologically a causal relationship between inhaled mold exposure and human illness in indoor environments, although associational relationships exist for some AHOs. For some types of illness, the term "insufficient" may mean that, although the data support such a conclusion, there are not enough data for the reviewers to reach a conclusion of "cause" or "association" for a particular AHO. Variations in study design and methodology, the complexity of molds and their FCs, a lack of standardized procedures for environmental assessments of mold and moisture, and other factors complicate the identification of potential relationships between mold exposure and AHOs. When methodologic confounders have been addressed more adequately, studies have been able more often to demonstrate strong relationships for some associations, such as the causal relationship of *Alternaria* to asthma. As in the case of hypersensitivity mechanisms, medical practitioners, including allergists, often operationally treat children who have illnesses that may be "associated" with or "caused" by mold exposure as if the relationship were causal, in the absence of an established "causal" relationship by strict epidemiologic criteria. Such is the case for most hypersensitivity disorders and most molds. As allergens, molds seem to act like other allergens in the diseases they cause, the medical evaluation they require for diagnosis, and the treatment that is effective.

It is clear that, to date, little evidence exists to support the conclusion that mold is responsible for some AHOs for which it is alleged to be the cause. Among the associations for which there is little evidence are toxic injuries from inhalation of mycotoxins in nonoccupational settings, systemic infection with *Candida* in immunocompetent hosts causing multiorgan system disease, and hypersensitivity to mold causing a rapid-onset cascade of neurocognitive symptoms. The relationships, or lack thereof, of cause and effect or association between mold and specific AHOs should become more evident with future investigations. That possibility exists only if the confounding factors noted previously are addressed adequately (eg, by larger subject populations and additional longitudinal studies).

There is the category of "indeterminate mechanisms." Even though it is not known exactly how dampness or mold produces some AHOs, there seems to be at least sufficient evidence for an association (Box 2) [6].

As discussed in this article, excessive moisture facilitates the growth or accumulation of various nonfungal microbial agents, insects, and rodents, all of which can result in AHOs similar to those from mold. The literature supporting other mold-related components, such as MVOCs and β-1,

Box 2. Summary of findings regarding the association between health outcomes and the presence of mold or other agents in damp indoor environments[1]

Sufficient evidence of a causal relationship
No outcomes met this definition

Sufficient evidence of an association
Upper respiratory tract (nasal and throat) symptoms
Asthma symptoms in sensitized asthmatic persons
Hypersensitivity pneumonitis in susceptible persons[2]
Wheeze
Cough

Limited or suggestive evidence of an association
Lower respiratory illness in otherwise-healthy children

Inadequate or insufficient evidence to determine whether an association exists
Dyspnea (shortness of breath)
Airflow obstruction (in otherwise-healthy persons)
Mucous membrane irritation syndrome
Chronic obstructive pulmonary disease
Inhalation fevers (nonoccupational exposures)
Lower respiratory illness in otherwise-healthy adults
Rheumatologic and other immune diseases
Acute idiopathic pulmonary hemorrhage in infants
Skin symptoms
Asthma development
Gastrointestinal tract problems
Fatigue
Neuropsychiatric symptoms
Cancer
Reproductive effects

---

[1] These conclusions are not applicable to immunocompromised persons, who are at increased risk for fungal colonization or opportunistic infections.
[2] For mold or bacteria in damp indoor environments.
Data from The Institute of Medicine of the National Academies. Damp indoor spaces and health. Washington, DC: The National Academies Press; 2004. p. 10.

3-D-glucan, as capable of producing AHOs is presently insufficient for the assignation of cause or even association. Nonmicrobial VOCs, however, have been shown to cause irritant effects by activating irritant receptors in the conjunctivae and airways.

Reservoirs of fungal growth can be found outdoors and, frequently, indoors. Exposure requires the FCs to get from the reservoir to the individual, and the amount of exposure depends on concentration and duration of expsoure. A high priority always should be assigned to the removal of reservoirs of mold in locations where a child might be exposed, even in the absence of any mold-related health problems. The required next step is to address and, if possible, eliminate the sources of excessive moisture producing those reservoirs. The interpretation of environmental data with a critical and knowing eye and the evaluation and treatment of children who have health problems that could be related to mold exposure are complex. A clinician who is unsure of the data, what to do with the data, or how to evaluate or treat a child who has a possible mold-related health problem should seek assistance from someone who has expertise in this type of environmental assessment or in the relevant pathophysiologic mechanisms of mold-induced injury.

References

[1] Spengler J, Neas L, Nakai S, et al. Respiratory symptoms and housing characteristics. Indoor Air 1994;4:72–82.
[2] Nevalainen A, Seuri M. Of microbes and men. Indoor Air 2005;15(Suppl 9):58–64.
[3] Portnoy J, Kwak K, Dowling P, et al. Health effects of indoor fungi. Ann Allergy 2005;94: 313–20.
[4] Fung F, Hughson W. Health effects of indoor fungal bioaerosol exposure. Appl Occup Environ Hyg 2003;18:535–44.
[5] Bush R, Portnoy J, Saxon A, et al. The medical effects of mold exposure. J Allergy Clin Immunol 2006;117(2):326–33.
[6] Institute of Medicine of the National Academies. Damp indoor spaces and health. Washington, DC: The National Academies Press; 2004.
[7] Kuhn D, Ghannoum M. Indoor mold, toxigenic fungi, and *Stachybotrys Chartarum*: infectious disease perspective. Clin Microbiol Rev 2003;16(1):144–72.
[8] Horner W, Helbling A, Salvaggio J, et al. Fungal allergens. Clin Microbiol Rev 1995;8(2): 161–79.
[9] Taskinen T, Hyvarinen A, Meklin T, et al. Asthma and respiratory infections in school children with special reference to moisture and mold problems in the school. Acta Paediatr 1999;88:1373–9.
[10] Halonen M, Stern D, Wright A, et al. *Alternaria* as a major allergen for asthma in children raised in a desert environment. Am J Respir Crit Care Med 1997;155:1356–61.
[11] O'Connor G, Walter M, Mitchell H, et al. Airborne fungi in the homes of children with asthma in low-income urban communities: the Inner-City Asthma Study. J Allergy Clin Immunol 2004;114:599–606.
[12] Eggleston P, Rosenstreich D, Lynn H, et al. Relationship of indoor allergen exposure to skin test sensitivity in inner-city children with asthma. J Allergy Clin Immunol 1998;102: 563–70.

[13] Arbes S, Gergen P, Elliott L, et al. Prevalences of positive skin test responses to 10 common allergens in the US population: results from the Third National Health and Nutrition Examination Survey. J Allergy Clin Immunol 2005;116:377–83.

[14] Bush R, Prochnau J. *Alternaria*-induced asthma. J Allergy Clin Immunol 2004;113:227–34.

[15] Bush R, Portnoy J. The role and abatement of fungal allergens in allergic diseases. J Allergy Clin Immunol 2001;107:S430–40.

[16] Bobbitt R, Crandall M, Venkataraman A, et al. Characterization of a population presenting with suspected mold-related health effects. Ann Allergy 2005;94:39–44.

[17] Blackley C. Experimental research on the cause and nature of *Catarrhus Aesitivus* (hay fever or hay asthma). London: Bailliere, Tindal and Cox; 1873. [revised edition, London, Dawson Pall Mall, 1959].

[18] Cantani V, Ciaschi V. Epidemiology of *Alternaria alternata* allergy: a prospective study of 6840 Italian asthmatic children. Eur Rev Med Pharmacol Sci 2004;8:289–94.

[19] Nelson H, Szefler S, Jacobs J, et al. The relationships among environmental allergen sensitization, allergen exposure, pulmonary function, and bronchial hyperresponsiveness in the Childhood Asthma Management Program. J Allergy Clin Immunol 1999;104: 775–85.

[20] Perzanowski M, Sporik R, Squillace S, et al. Association of sensitization to *Alternaria* allergens with asthma among school-age children. J Allergy Clin Immunol 1998;101:626–32.

[21] Sanchez H, Bush R. A review of *Alternaria alternata* sensitivity. Rev Iberoam Micol 2001; 18:56–9.

[22] O'Hollaren MT, Yunginger JW, Offord KP, et al. Exposure to an aeroallergen as a possible precipitating factor in respiratory arrest in young patients with asthma. N Engl J Med 1991; 324(6):359–63.

[23] Nilsson D, Aas K. Immunological specificity and correlation of diagnostic tests for bronchial allergy to *Cladosporium herbarum*. Acta Paediatr Scand 1976;65:33–8.

[24] Zock J, Jarvis D, Luczynska C, et al. Housing characteristics, reported mold exposure, and asthma in the European Community Respiratory Health Survey. J Allergy Clin Immunol 2002;110:285–92.

[25] Malling H, Dreborg S, Weeke B. Diagnosis and immunotherapy of mold allergy. III. Allergy 1986;41:507–19.

[26] Dreborg S, Agrell B, Foucard T, et al. A double-blind, multicenter immunotherapy trial in children using a purified and standardized Cladosporium preparation. Allergy 1986;41: 131–40.

[27] Malling H, Dreborg S, Weeke B. Diagnosis and immunotherapy of mould allergy. VI. IgE-mediated parameters during a one-year placebo-controlled study of immunotherapy with *Cladosporium*. Allergy 1987;42(4):305–14.

[28] Horst M, Hejjaoui A, Horst V, et al. Double-blind, placebo-controlled rush immunotherapy with a standardized *Alternaria* extract. J Allergy Clin Immunol 1990;85:460–72.

[29] Cantani A, Businco E, Maglio A. Alternaria allergy: a three-year controlled study in children treated with immunotherapy. Allergol Immunopathol (Madr) 1988;16(1):1–4.

[30] Bernardis P, Agnoletto M, Puccinelli P, et al. Injective versus sublingual immunotherapy in *Alternaria tenuis* allergic patients. J Investig Allergol Clin Immunol 1996;6(1):55–62.

[31] Kidon I, See Y, Goh A, et al. Aeroallergen sensitization in pediatric allergic rhinitis in Singapore: is air-conditioning a factor in the tropics? Pediatr Allergy Immunol 2004;15: 340–3.

[32] Volovitz B, Osur SL, Bernstein JM, et al. Leukotriene C4 release in upper respiratory mucosa during natural exposure to ragweed in ragweed-sensitive children. J Allergy Clin Immunol 1988;82(3 Pt 1):414–8.

[33] Stark P, Celedon J, Chew G, et al. Fungal levels in the home and allergic rhinitis by 5 years of age. Environ Health Perspect 2005;113:1405–9.

[34] Huang S-W, Giannoni C. The risk of adenoid hypertrophy in children with allergic rhinitis. Ann Allergy Asthma Immunol 2001;87:350–5.

[35] Huang SW. The risk of sinusitis in children with allergic rhinitis. Allergy Asthma Proc 2000; 21(2):85–8.

[36] Wilken JA, Berkowitz R, Kane R. Decrements in vigilance and cognitive functioning associated with ragweed-induced allergic rhinitis. Ann Allergy Asthma Immunol 2002;89(4): 372–80.

[37] Dunleavy RA, Baade LE. Neuropsychological correlates of severe asthma in children 9–14 years old. J Consult Clin Psychol 1980;48(2):214–9.

[38] Bender BG. Cognitive effects of allergic rhinitis and its treatment. Immunol Allergy Clin North Am 2005;25(2):301–12, [vi–vii].

[39] Dykewicz MS, Fineman S. Executive summary of joint task force practice parameters on diagnosis and management of rhinitis. Ann Allergy Asthma Immunol 1998;81(5 Pt 2): 463–8.

[40] Wananukul S, Huiprasert P, Pongprasit P. Eczematous skin reaction from patch testing with aeroallergens in atopic children without atopic dermatitis. Pediatr Dermatol 1993; 10(3):209–13.

[41] Clark R, Adinoff A. Aeroallergen contact can exacerbate atopic dermatitis: patch tests as a diagnostic tool. J Am Acad Dermatol 1989;21:863–9.

[42] Sampson H. The role of "allergy" in atopic dermatitis. Clin Rev Allergy 1986;4:125–38.

[43] Drouet M, Bouillaud E. Anaphylactic reaction to *Aspergillus*. Allerg Immunol (Paris) 1996; 28(3):88–9.

[44] Torricelli R, Johansson S, Withrich B. Ingestive and inhalative allergy to the mushroom *Boletus edulis*. Allergy 1997;52(7):747–51.

[45] Maibach H. Contact urticaria syndrome from mold on salami casing. Contact Derm 1995; 32(2):120–1.

[46] Turner E, Greenberger PA, Sider M. Complexities of establishing an early diagnosis of allergic bronchopulmonary aspergillosis in children. Allergy Proc 1989;10(1):63–9.

[47] McCarthy D, Pepys J. Allergic broncho-pulmonary aspergillosis. Clinical immunology: (2) skin, nasal and bronchial tests. Clin Allergy 1971;1:415–32.

[48] Greenberger P, et al. Allergic bronchopulmonary aspergillosis. In: Adkinson N Jr, Yunginger J, Busse W, editors. Middleton's allergy principles & practice, vol 2. 6th edition. Philadelphia: Mosby; 2003. p. 1353–71.

[49] Knutsen A, Blakeslee N, Manoj R, et al. Allergic bronchopulmonary aspergillosis in a patient with cystic fibrosis: diagnostic criteria when the IgE level is less than 500 IU/ml. Ann Allergy 2005;95:488–93.

[50] Laufer P, Fink J, Bruns W, et al. Allergic bronchopulmonary aspergillosis in cystic fibrosis. J Allergy Clin Immunol 1984;73(1 pt 1):44–8.

[51] Greenberger PA, Patterson R. Allergic bronchopulmonary aspergillosis and the evaluation of the patient with asthma. J Allergy Clin Immunol 1988;81(4):646–50.

[52] Imbeau S, Cohen M, Reed C. Allergic bronchopulmonary aspergillosis in infants. Am J Dis Child 1977;131:1127–30.

[53] Saini S, Boas S, Jerah A, et al. Allergic bronchopulmonary mycosis to *Fusarium vasinfectum* in a child. Ann Allergy 1998;80:377–80.

[54] Donnelly S, McLaughlin H, Brendin C. Period prevalence of allergic bronchopulmonary mycosis in a regional hospital outpatient population in Ireland 1985–88. Ir J Med Sci 1991;160(9):288–90.

[55] Katzenstein A, Sale S, Greenberger PA. Allergic Aspergillus sinusitis: a newly recognized form of sinusitis. J Allergy Clin Immunol 1983;72(1):89–93.

[56] Kupferberg S, Bent J. Allergic fungal sinusitis in the pediatric population. Arch Otolaryngol Head Neck Surg 1996;122:1381–4.

[57] deShazo R, Swain R. Diagnostic criteria for allergic fungal sinusitis. J Allergy Clin Immunol 1995;96(1):24–35.

[58] Marple BF. Allergic fungal rhinosinusitis: current theories and management strategies. Laryngoscope 2001;111(6):1006–19.

[59] Schubert M. Medical treatment of allergic fungal sinusitis. Ann Allergy 2000;85:90–101.
[60] McClay J, Marple B. Allergic fungal sinusitis. 2006. Available at: http://www.emedicine. com/ent/topic510.htm.
[61] McClay J, Marple B, Kapadia L, et al. Clinical presentation of allergic fungal sinusitis in children. Laryngoscope 2002;112:565–9.
[62] Chhabra A, Handa KK, Chakrabarti A, et al. Allergic fungal sinusitis: clinicopathological characteristics. Mycoses 1996;39(11–12):437–41.
[63] Muntz H. Allergic fungal sinusitis in children. Otolaryngol Clin North Am 1996;29(1): 185–92.
[64] Fan L. Hypersensitivity pneumonitis in children. Curr Opin Pediatr 2002;14:323–6.
[65] Greenberger PA. Mold-induced hypersensitivity pneumonitis. Allergy Asthma Proc 2004; 25(4):219–23.
[66] Chiron C, Gaultier C, Boule M, et al. Lung function in children with hypersensitivity pneumonitis. Eur J Respir Dis 1984;65:79–91.
[67] Fink JN, Schlueter DP, Sosman AJ, et al. Clinical survey of pigeon breeders. Chest 1972; 62(3):277–81.
[68] Ratjen F, Costabel U, Griese M, et al. Bronchoalveolar lavage fluid findings in children with hypersensitivity pneumonitis. Eur Respir J 2003;21:144–8.
[69] Aebischer CC, Frey U, Schoni MH. Hypersensitivity pneumonitis in a five-year-old boy: an unusual antigen source. Pediatr Pulmonol 2002;33(1):77–8.
[70] O'Connell EJ, Zora JA, Gillespie DN, et al. Childhood hypersensitivity pneumonitis (farmer's lung): four cases in siblings with long-term follow-up. J Pediatr 1989;114(6): 995–7.
[71] Jacobs R, Thorner R, Holcomb J, et al. Hypersensitivity pneumonitis caused by *Cladosporium* in an enclosed hot-tub area. Ann Intern Med 1986;105(2):204–6.
[72] Hogan MB, Patterson R, Pore RS, et al. Basement shower hypersensitivity pneumonitis secondary to *Epicoccum nigrum*. Chest 1996;110(3):854–6.
[73] Lee S-K, Kim S-S, Nahm D-H, et al. Hypersensitivity pneumonitis caused by *Fusarium napiforme* in a home environment. Allergy 2000;55:1190–3.
[74] Sugiyama K, Mukae H, Ishii H, et al. Familial summer-type hypersensitivity pneumonitis— case report and review of literature. Nihon Kokyuki Gakkai Zasshi 2005;43(11):683–8.
[75] Iyori J, Kawamura K, Seo K. Summer-type hypersensitivity pneumonitis in a child. Acta Paediatr Jpn 1991;33(4):488–91.
[76] Roeder A, Kirschning CJ, Rupec RA, et al. Toll-like receptors and innate antifungal responses. Trends Microbiol 2004;12(1):44–9.
[77] Roeder A, Kirschning CJ, Rupec RA, et al. Toll-like receptors as key mediators in innate antifungal immunity. Med Mycol 2004;42(6):485–98.
[78] Marodi L. Innate cellular immune responses in newborns. Clin Immunol 2006;118(2–3): 137–44.
[79] Wan G-H, Li C-S, Guo S-P, et al. An airborne mold-derived product, β-1,3-D-glucan, potentiates airway allergic responses. Eur J Immunol 1999;29:2491–7.
[80] Hohl T, Van Epps H, Rivera A, et al. *Aspergillus fumigatus* triggers inflammatory responses by stage-specific β-glucan display. PLos Pathog 2005;1:232–40.
[81] Fogelmark B, Goto H, Yuasa K, et al. Acute pulmonary toxicity of inhaled β -1,3-glucan and endotoxin. Agents Actions 1992;35(1–2):50–6.
[82] Holt P. Potential role of environmental factors in the etiology and pathogenesis of atopy: a working model. Environ Health Perspect 1999;107(Suppl 3):485–7.
[83] Thorn J, Beijer L, Rylander R. Effects after inhalation of $(1 \rightarrow 3)$- β - D-glucan in healthy humans. Mediators Inflamm 2001;10:173–8.
[84] Beijer L, Thorn J, Rylander R. Effects after inhalation of $(1 \rightarrow 3)$ - β - D - glucan and relation to mould exposure in the home. Mediators Inflamm 2002;11(3):149–53.
[85] Beijer L, Thorn J, Rylander R. Mould exposure at home relates to inflammatory markers in blood. Eur Respir J 2003;21:317–92.

[86] Hirvonen MR, Huttunen K, Roponen M. Bacterial strains from moldy buildings are highly potent inducers of inflammatory and cytotoxic effects. Indoor Air 2005;15(Suppl 9): 65–70.

[87] Douwes J. (1→3)-β-D-glucans and respiratory health: a review of the scientific evidence. Indoor Air 2005;15:160–9.

[88] Kheradmand F, Kiss A, Xu J, et al. A protease-activated pathway underlying Th cell type 2 activation and allergic lung disease. J Immunol 2002;169(10):5904–11.

[89] Kauffman HF, Tomee JF, van de Riet MA, et al. Protease-dependent activation of epithelial cells by fungal allergens leads to morphologic changes and cytokine production. J Allergy Clin Immunol 2000;105(6 Pt 1):1185–93.

[90] Johanning E, Biagini R, Hull D, et al. Health and immunology study following exposure to toxigenic fungi (Stachybotrys chartarum) in a water-damaged office environment. Int Arch Occup Environ Health 1996;68(4):207–18.

[91] Hodgson MJ, Morey P, Leung WY, et al. Building-associated pulmonary disease from exposure to Stachybotrys chartarum and Aspergillus versicolor. J Occup Environ Med 1998;40(3):241–9.

[92] Burge HA. Fungi: toxic killers or unavoidable nuisances? Ann Allergy Asthma Immunol 2001;87(6 Suppl 3):52–6.

[93] Etzel RA. Mycotoxins. JAMA 2002;287(4):425–7.

[94] Robbins CA, Swenson LJ, Nealley ML, et al. Health effects of mycotoxins in indoor air: a critical review. Appl Occup Environ Hyg 2000;15(10):773–84.

[95] Page EH, Trout DB. The role of Stachybotrys mycotoxins in building-related illness. AIHAJ 2001;62(5):644–8.

[96] Hardin BD, Kelman BJ, Saxon A. Adverse human health effects associated with molds in the indoor environment. J Occup Environ Med 2003;45(5):470–8.

[97] Montalbano M, Lemanske R. Infections and asthma in children. Curr Opin Pediatr 2002; 14(3):334–7.

[98] Kelman BJ, Robbins CA, Swenson LJ, et al. Risk from inhaled mycotoxins in indoor office and residential environments. Int J Toxicol 2004;23(1):3–10.

[99] Jarvis BB, Miller JD. Mycotoxins as harmful indoor air contaminants. Appl Microbiol Biotechnol 2005;66(4):367–72.

[100] Etzel RA, Montana E, Sorenson WG, et al. Acute pulmonary hemorrhage in infants associated with exposure to Stachybotrys atra and other fungi. Arch Pediatr Adolesc Med 1998;152(8):757–62.

[101] Centers for Disease Control. Update: pulmonary hemorrhage/hemosiderosis among infants—Cleveland, Ohio, 1993–1996. MMWR Morb Mortal Wkly Rep 1997;46(2):33–5.

[102] Dearborn DG, Smith PG, Dahms BB, et al. Clinical profile of 30 infants with acute pulmonary hemorrhage in Cleveland. Pediatrics 2002;110(3):627–37.

[103] Elidemir O, Colasurdo GN, Rossmann SN, et al. Isolation of Stachybotrys from the lung of a child with pulmonary hemosiderosis. Pediatrics 1999;104(4 Pt 1):964–6.

[104] Etzel RA. Stachybotrys. Curr Opin Pediatr 2003;15(1):103–6.

[105] Yike I, Dearborn DG. Pulmonary effects of Stachybotrys chartarum in animal studies. Adv Appl Microbiol 2004;55:241–73.

[106] Yike I, Rand TG, Dearborn DG. Acute inflammatory responses to Stachybotrys chartarum in the lungs of infant rats: time course and possible mechanisms. Toxicol Sci 2005;84(2): 408–17.

[107] Fung F, Clark RF. Health effects of mycotoxins: a toxicological overview. J Toxicol Clin Toxicol 2004;42(2):217–34.

[108] Belson MG, Schier JG, Patel MM. Case definitions for chemical poisoning. MMWR Recomm Rep 2005;54(RR-1):1–24.

[109] Trout DB, Seltzer JM, Page EH, et al. Clinical use of immunoassays in assessing exposure to fungi and potential health effects related to fungal exposure. Ann Allergy Asthma Immunol 2004;92(5):483–91 [quiz: 492–4, 575].

332   SELTZER & FEDORUK

[110] Gilbert J, Brereton P, MacDonald S. Assessment of dietary exposure to ochratoxin A in the UK using a duplicate diet approach and analysis of urine and plasma samples. Food Addit Contam 2001;18(12):1088–93.
[111] Meky FA, Turner PC, Ashcroft AE, et al. Development of a urinary biomarker of human exposure to deoxynivalenol. Food Chem Toxicol 2003;41(2):265–73.
[112] Von Essen S, Robbins RA, Thompson AB, et al. Organic dust toxic syndrome: an acute febrile reaction to organic dust exposure distinct from hypersensitivity pneumonitis. J Toxicol Clin Toxicol 1990;28(4):389–420.
[113] Rask-Andersen A. Organic dust toxic syndrome among farmers. Br J Ind Med 1989;46(4):233–8.
[114] Brinton WT, Vastbinder EE, Greene JW, et al. An outbreak of organic dust toxic syndrome in a college fraternity. JAMA 1987;258(9):1210–2.
[115] Latge JP, Calderone R. Host-microbe interactions: fungi invasive human fungal opportunistic infections. Curr Opin Microbiol 2002;5(4):355–8.
[116] Groll AH, Walsh TJ. Uncommon opportunistic fungi: new nosocomial threats. Clin Microbiol Infect 2001;7(Suppl 2):8–24.
[117] Weems JJ Jr, Davis BJ, Tablan OC, et al. Construction activity: an independent risk factor for invasive aspergillosis and zygomycosis in patients with hematologic malignancy. Infect Control 1987;8(2):71–5.
[118] Perraud M, Piens MA, Nicoloyannis N, et al. Invasive nosocomial pulmonary aspergillosis: risk factors and hospital building works. Epidemiol Infect 1987;99(2):407–12.
[119] Krasinski K, Holzman RS, Hanna B, et al. Nosocomial fungal infection during hospital renovation. Infect Control 1985;6(7):278–82.
[120] Buffington J, Reporter R, Lasker BA, et al. Investigation of an epidemic of invasive aspergillosis: utility of molecular typing with the use of random amplified polymorphic DNA probes. Pediatr Infect Dis J 1994;13(5):386–93.
[121] Sehulster L, Chinn RY. Guidelines for environmental infection control in health-care facilities. Recommendations of CDC and the Healthcare Infection Control Practices Advisory Committee (HICPAC). MMWR Recomm Rep 2003;52(RR-10):1–42.
[122] Shusterman D. Toxicology of nasal irritants. Curr Allergy Asthma Rep 2003;3:258–65.
[123] Veronesi B, Oortgiesen M. Neurogenic inflammation and particulate matter (PM) air pollutants. Neurotoxicology 2001;22:795–810.
[124] Widdicombe J. Afferent receptors in the airways and cough. Respir Physiol 1998;114:5–15.
[125] Cometto-Muniz J, Cain W. Physicochemical determinants and functional properties of the senses of irritation and smell. In: Gammage R, Berven B, editors. Indoor air and human health. 2nd edition. New York: CRC Press; 1996. p. 53–65.
[126] Nilsson A, Kihlstrom E, Lagesson V, et al. Microorganisms and volatile organic compounds in airborne dust from damp residences. Indoor Air 2004;14:74–82.
[127] Saijo Y, Kishi R, Sata F, et al. Symptoms in relation to chemicals and dampness in newly built dwellings. Int Arch Occup Environ Health 2004;77:461–70.
[128] Laumbach R, Kipen H. Bioaerosols and sick building syndrome: particles, inflammation, and allergy. Curr Opin Allergy Clin Immunol 2005;5:135–9.
[129] Straus D, Cooley J, Wong W, et al. Studies on the role of fungi in sick building syndrome. Arch Environ Health 2003;58(8):475–8.
[130] Wilson S, Straus D. The presence of fungi associated with sick building syndrome in North American zoological institutions. J Zoo Wildl Med 2002;33(4):322–7.
[131] Cooley J, Wong W, Jumper C, et al. Correlation between the prevalence of certain fungi and sick building syndrome. Occup Environ Med 1998;55:579–84.
[132] Baldo JV, Ahmad L, Ruff R. Neuropsychological performance of patients following mold exposure. Appl Neuropsychol 2002;9(4):193–202.
[133] Handal G, Leiner MA, Cabrera M, et al. Children symptoms before and after knowing about an indoor fungal contamination. Indoor Air 2004;14(2):87–91.
[134] Khalili B, Bardana E. International mold toxicity: fact or fiction? A clinical review of 50 cases. Ann Allergy 2005;95:239–46.

[135] Khalili B, Montanaro M, Bardana E. Indoor mold and your patient's health: from suspicion to confirmation. J Respir Dis 2005;26(120):520–5.

[136] Platt S, Martin C, Hunt S, et al. Damp housing, mould growth and symptomatic health state. Br Med J 1989;298:1673–8.

[137] Dales R, Zwanenberg H, Burnett R, et al. Respiratory health effects of home dampness and molds among Canadian children. Am J Epidemiol 1991;134:196–203.

[138] Brunekreef B, Dockery D, Speizer F, et al. Home dampness and respiratory morbidity in children. Am Rev Respir Dis 1989;140:1363–7.

[139] Hynes P, Brugge D, Osgood N, et al. Investigations into the indoor environment and respiratory health in Boston public housing. Rev Environ Health 2004;19(3–4):271–89.

[140] Horner W. The damp building effect: understanding needed, not more debate. Ann Allergy 2005;94:213–5.

[141] Dekker C, Dales R, Bartlett S, et al. Childhood asthma and the indoor environment. Chest 1991;100:922–6.

[142] Li C-S, Hsu L-Y. Home dampness and childhood respiratory symptoms in a subtropical climate. Arch Environ Health 1996;51(1):42–6.

[143] Yang C-Y, Cheng M-F, Tsai S-S, et al. Effects of indoor environmental factors on risk for acute otitis media in a subtropical area. J Toxicol Environ Health A 1999;56:111–9.

[144] Strachan D, Elton R. Relationship between respiratory morbidity in children and the home environment. Fam Pract 1986;3(3):137–42.

[145] Jedrychowski W, Flak E. Separate and combined effects of the outdoor and indoor air quality on chronic respiratory symptoms adjusted for allergy among preadolescent children. Int J Occup Med Environ Health 1998;11(1):19–35.

[146] Peat JK, Dickerson J, Li J. Effects of damp and mould in the home on respiratory health: a review of the literature. Allergy 1998;53(2):120–8.

[147] Jaakkola J, Jaakkola N, Ruotsalainen R. Home dampness and molds as determinants of respiratory symptoms and asthma in pre-school children. J Expo Anal Environ Epidemiol 1993;3(Suppl 1):129–42.

[148] Strachan D, Sanders C. Damp housing and childhood asthma; respiratory effects of indoor air and temperature and relative humidity. J Epidemiol Community Health 1989;43:7–14.

[149] Bornehag C, Blomquist G, Gyntelberg F, et al. Dampness in buildings and health. Indoor Air 2001;11:72–86.

[150] Santilli J. Health effects of mold exposure in public schools. Curr Allergy Asthma Rep 2002; 2:460–7.

[151] Rylander R, Norrhall M, Engdahl U, et al. Airways inflammation, atopy, and (1→3)-β-D-glucan. Am J Respir Crit Care Med 1998;158:1685–7.

[152] Meklin T, Husman T, Vepsalainen M, et al. Indoor air microbes and respiratory symptoms of children in moisture damaged and reference schools. Indoor Air 2002;12:175–83.

[153] Meklin T, Potus T, Pekkanen J, et al. Effects of moisture-damage repairs on microbial exposure and symptoms in schoolchildren. Indoor Air 2005;15(Suppl 10):40–7.

[154] Savilahti R, Uitti J, Laippala P, et al. Respiratory morbidity among children following renovation of a water-damaged school. Arch Environ Health 2000;55(6):405–10.

[155] Savilahti R, Uitti J, Roto P, et al. Increased prevalence of atopy among children exposed to mold in a school building. Allergy 2001;56(2):175–9.

[156] Meyer H, Wurtz H, Suadicani P, et al. Molds in floor dust and building-related symptoms in adolescent school children. Indoor Air 2004;14:65–72.

[157] Meyer H, Wurtz H, Suadicani P, et al. Molds in floor dust and building-related symptoms among adolescent school children: a problem for boys only? Indoor Air 2005;15(Suppl 10): 17–24.

[158] Scheel C, Rosing W, Farone A. Possible sources of sick building syndrome in a Tennessee middle school. Arch Environ Health 2001;56(5):413–9.

[159] Bartlett K, Kennedy S, Brauer M, et al. Evaluation and a predictive model of airborne fungal concentrations in school classrooms. Ann Occup Hyg 2004;48(6):547–54.

ELSEVIER
SAUNDERS

Pediatr Clin N Am
54 (2007) 335–350

PEDIATRIC CLINICS
OF NORTH AMERICA

Global Pediatric Environmental Health

Tee L. Guidotti, MD, MPH, DABT[a,b,*],
Benjamin A. Gitterman, MD, FAAP[b,c]

[a]*Department of Environmental and Occupational Health, School of Public Health
and Health Services, George Washington University Medical Center,
2100 M Street, NW, Suite 203, Washington, DC 20052, USA*
[b]*Mid-Atlantic Center for Children's Health and the Environment, Washington, DC, USA*
[c]*Children's National Medical Center and George Washington University School
of Medicine and Health Sciences, Washington, DC, USA*

According to the World Health Organization (WHO), at least 3 million children die each year from causes related to the environment. Most of these deaths are caused by diarrhea and result from poor sanitation and water quality. Most of the remaining cases are caused by malaria, an infectious disease resulting from an environment that supports the breeding and proliferation of the mosquito vector. Beyond these fatal cases, 40% of the global burden of environmental disease falls on the world's 2.3 billion children [1].

In 2004, the World Health Organization published the Atlas of Children's Environmental Health and the Environment [2]. This valuable resource maps the distribution of environmental health problems on a large scale. It vividly demonstrates that there are two world regimes as far as the health of children are concerned. Developed countries report as the most common problems ambient (outdoor) air pollution and lead. Developing countries (and Russia, outside the major western cities) have a wider range of common problems, including childhood injuries; indoor air pollution (caused by burning of biomass); infectious disease; and poor sanitation with unsafe water. This is a discouraging list because it would have been the same 50 years ago, and is even worse today in that air pollution was not as appreciated then as a serious health hazard and malaria was less prevalent in many countries of sub-Saharan Africa. The Atlas demonstrates the close link between economic development and achievement of a less threatening

* Corresponding author. Department of Environmental and Occupational Health, School of Public Health and Health Services, George Washington University Medical Center, 2100 M Street, NW, Suite 203, Washington, DC 20052.

E-mail address: eohtlg@gwumc.edu (T.L. Guidotti).

0031-3955/07/$ - see front matter © 2007 Elsevier Inc. All rights reserved.
doi:10.1016/j.pcl.2007.03.002
pediatric.theclinics.com

environment for children. Less threatening, however, does not necessarily mean safe and healthy in absolute terms.

The Atlas conceals in its high-level aggregation another important truth about hazards that threaten children. Children's environmental health is a global problem, not an issue confined to developing countries. Hazards to the health of children are present everywhere people live, whether the society is developed or developing. The frequency and severity of the hazard may change but risks from injury, lead, air pollution, poor sanitation, and preventable infectious disease are universal. Many affluent societies, including North America [1], have failed to control common risks, such as vehicular injury and air pollution. Almost all affluent societies have within them pockets of poverty or less-developed regions where poverty-related environmental health problems continue to threaten the health of children.

Children are uniquely vulnerable to environmental health problems. As noted elsewhere in this issue, they are biologically more susceptible and exposed to the most widespread environmental hazards. The unique vulnerability of children arises, however, particularly from social factors. Children cannot take care of themselves. They rely on a functioning society and infrastructure to protect them, and when society fails them, children suffer more than adults. Even in societies in which there is a functioning child welfare system that protects children and a functioning public health system that looks after the health of its people, neglect, abuse or ignorance at the level of the family may place children at risk in their own community.

Children are vulnerable to environmental exposure around the world, in both developed and developing societies. The threats to children's health are generally greater in societies that are in the transition from agrarian to industrialized economies, however, in which potential toxic exposures have been introduced but protection is lacking and poverty or ignorance forces unsafe practices at work or home, and may include the child in the workforce.

This article presents an overview of the major issues in global pediatric environmental health, particularly in developing countries. Although hardly comprehensive, it touches on parallels to issues in the developed world and to the unique social and economic situations that place children in these settings at special risk. These risks might be difficult to imagine in the setting of a developed country, yet they significantly affect the health and well-being of children in settings different than those of most readers of this article.

Hazards specific to children

Lead

Acute lead poisoning, as a syndrome of symptoms and signs of toxic effects in the individual, has become rare in the United States. Recent studies confirm that the primary risk continues to arise from ingestion of lead paint chips and dust and from other, less common, but relatively highly concentrated sources, such as lead-containing jewelry and ceramics. A rare, fatal case of domestic lead poisoning occurred in 2006 when a child in Minneapolis ingested a lead-containing ornament, manufactured overseas, which was used as decoration on a popular sports shoe [3]. As acute and chronic symptomatic lead poisoning has become less common, control of chronic lead toxicity at lower exposure levels has taken center stage in developed countries, such as the United States.

Acute and chronic lead poisoning remains a problem in many developing countries, including India, where sources of exposure at high levels include lead paint, leaded gasoline, and lead-containing medicaments and cosmetics [4]. Although much less common, individual cases of lead poisoning in children remain devastating, with a high risk of residual mental impairment.

Chronic toxicity at or near the current WHO and Centers for Disease Control and Prevention "level of concern" in blood of 10 µg/dL, which in 1992 was thought to be protective, has remained a problem in many countries that continue to use leaded gasoline, such as South Africa [5], Bangladesh [6], and Indonesia [7]. It has been demonstrated to be at high prevalence among children adopted by American families, especially from China [8].

In the United States, the mean level of blood lead in children is dropping steadily, but the recognition of neurobehavioral effects below the level of concern has spurred interest in a more comprehensive strategy for lead elimination [9].

When sources are widely dispersed, as in many developing countries, as has been described in Africa [10], this may be very difficult and compliance may be poor, as documented in Latin America [11]. In some situations, as in the heavily lead-contaminated city of Kabwe, Zambia, it may seem impossible. Fortunately the elimination of leaded gasoline in many countries worldwide is actively under way and will substantially reduce exposure from that source.

Child labor

The large number of working preadolescent children in developing countries who are not going to school is a result of poverty, poorly developed educational systems, lack of or poorly enforced legislation, or lack of public awareness [12]. They have great vulnerability to the dangers and stress of such work, including physical, chemical, and psychologic risks. Of greatest concern are the conditions in which they work. Increased advocacy and protection of the rights of children are critical to their health and survival.

Dangerous work exposures are numerous. They may include pesticides during farm work, benzene during work at gasoline stations, lead at the time of vehicle repair, asbestos and silica during construction and maintenance work, and loud noise during manufacturing [13]. The potentials for injury are equally numerous, because children often work in mines, brick manufacture, quarries, marketplaces, rocketry manufacturing sites, agriculture, and domestic work [14]. Child labor is prevalent in rural and agricultural areas and the nature of many hazardous exposures is diverse. The lack of formal safety supervision or training of these children in issues of safety increases their risk exposure.

The emotional risk factors to a child are a result of the work environment. There may be an expectation that children help support the family, resulting in work at a young age, with long work hours. This can occur at home, on a farm, or in forced child labor. Slavery, sexual abuse, or prostitution may be prevalent. They may be abandoned or live on the street, and be further exploited. Children, even if physically capable of the work expected of them, may be emotionally immature, and unable to understand their own abilities to work safely. They may work lengthy days, resulting in exhaustion, poor judgment, and subsequent increased physical and emotional risks [15].

Pesticides

Acute pesticide exposure among children remains a risk in rural households, especially in tropical countries where families live in close proximity to agricultural chemicals and farming operations. Incidents of unintentional acute exposure are poorly documented in most developing countries but probably occur more often than in developing countries. Such incidents probably occur more often in the United States than in other developed countries, because of risks experienced by the large migrant farm worker population. The extent to which acute toxicity occurs inadvertently as a result of deliberate exposure in homes for pest control is also unknown, but that it may be a problem is suggested by the experience of methylparathion use in the United States South. Families had used this highly toxic pesticide to control cockroaches and other pests in their homes, resulting in a risk to children [16]. Similar incidents almost certainly happen elsewhere, but probably go unnoticed.

Environmental exposure to pesticides is intense and toxicologically significant in some developing countries. Depressed cholinesterase levels have been documented among children in Nicaragua living downstream from a crop-dusting airport [17]. Prolonged pesticide use, the development of pest species resistance, and exposure to residues may be of greater importance in settings with lesser controls and technology and with greater dependence on agriculture. Children may be often exposed to chlorpyrifos because of frequent indoor use. Accidental exposures may also be more frequent because of common use of unmarked receptacles, or those that are not safely stored because of poor supervision.

Persistent organic pollutants

Persistent organic pollutants (POPs) are halogenated but carbon-based chemicals, usually relatively simple but sometimes with complicated structures, that resist the natural mechanisms of catabolism in the environment and so remain unchanged for long periods. Most POPs are organochlorine pesticides, such as toxaphene, chlordane, DDT (dichloro-diphenyl-trichloroethane), mirex, aldrin, and dieldrin, all of which are no longer produced in developed countries or have very restricted uses. Other POPs include polychlorinated biphenyls, and chlorinated dibenzo-dioxins and furans. The polychlorinated biphenyls are no longer produced, and dioxins and furans are mostly found as unwanted contaminants of other chemical processes.

These compounds are lipophilic and so are found in greatest concentration in fatty organs, such as liver and adipose tissue, and organisms with extensive body fat, such as seals. Because they are refractory to the usual biochemical pathways of degradation in soil bacteria, mold, and in animal species, these compounds are also subject to bioconcentration and biomagnification, accumulating to greater concentrations in species with increasing trophic level. They migrate within the ecosystem depending on temperature, mobilized during warmer temperatures and condensing on surfaces during cold weather. Because of these phenomena, there has been a gradual accumulation of POPs in northern latitudes.

The greatest concern for toxicity to human beings has been dioxin-like metabolic effects, cancer risk, and endocrine-mimic activity. The best-documented effect to date, however, has been an inferred immune defect that is thought to be responsible for increased frequency of otitis media in Inuit children in the high Arctic, where ecologic fate and disposition pathways, steep food chains, and a lipid-rich diet have resulted in the highest exposure levels recorded.

In 1997, under the auspices of the United Nations, the Stockholm Convention on Persistent Organic Pollutants was introduced. Better known as the "POPs Treaty," this international agreement calls on the signatory nations to monitor, reduce, and ultimately eliminate designated POPs compounds from the environment, including unused stockpiles. The POPs Treaty has been generally effective and levels of POPs are declining throughout the world. It is considered one of the major success stories of environmental regulation on an international scale [18].

Fluoride

Fluoride is a naturally occurring trace element, in soil and water, and may also be present as a by-product of fertilizer and aluminum industries. Significant elevation of fluoride levels may occur in deep groundwater wells in high fluoride concentration areas reaching levels as great as 20 times the level in usual surface water. Fluoride may be present in coal, and is released during burning.

In generally accepted controlled doses, fluoride is beneficial in preventing or reducing the incidence of dental caries. At higher concentrations it causes fluorosis, of which the major sign is mottled discoloration of the teeth.

Fluorosis is not commonly seen in developed countries. Excess fluoride may result in dental, skeletal, and nonskeletal fluorosis. Dental fluorosis initially causes cosmetic discoloration of the teeth but may result in tooth decay if it is advanced. Skeletal fluorosis may result in deformities of the joints and extremities and subsequent crippling limitations in physical activity may occur [19].

It is believed that as many as 100 million persons may suffer from fluoride overexposure. In some areas of Africa and the Middle East, volcanic rock and sediment are naturally weathered, resulting in high concentrations of fluoride in deep groundwater. India, Mexico, China, and Bangladesh have naturally occurring high levels in groundwater [20].

Solutions are not simple. Changes in local water sources from deep groundwater wells to piped drinking water could help. The piped water itself, however, often contains inappropriate high levels of fluoride. Rainwater, when collected, might seem a logical alternative in some cases, but it may not be available all year long in very dry areas. Defluorination programs and technologies are not yet readily available to meet existing needs [21].

Endocrine disruptors

Endocrine disruptors are exogenous chemicals that mimic or modify the action of endogenous hormones and alter the normal functioning of the endocrine system. The term applies to substances that interfere with complex hormonal processes, such as thyroid hormone, insulin and androgen activity, estrogens, and the multiple hormonal interactions that result in puberty and development [22]. Potential adverse outcomes may be neurodevelopmental, neurobehavioral, reproductive, immune related, or cancer related. The primary route of exposure concern is ingestion and subsequent transplacental passage. This puts the embryo, fetus, and young child at risk. It is increasingly hypothesized (but not proved) that these exposures may be responsible for an increasing incidence of testicular cancer, doubling of the incidence of hypospadias, and the increasingly early onset of puberty in girls [22].

POPs remain in the environment, bioaccumulate along the food chain, and are a risk to human health. A list of persistent organic pollutants is previously enumerated. Although POPs are being phased out of use overall, they resist biodegradation and are insoluble in water. They are readily stored in human fat tissue where concentrations may be quite high. They may also be passed on in breast milk.

Additional chemical classes may be endocrine disruptors and raise concern. They include natural and synthetic hormones, plant constituents, pesticides, and compounds used in the plastic industry. They are widely dispersed in the environment, can be transported long distances, and are found in most regions of the world. Some persist, others are rapidly degraded [23].

POPS and other endocrine disruptors are toxic at high concentrations. Data are not yet available firmly to evaluate the effects of low-level chronic exposures. These outcomes may also be dependent on a sophisticated analysis of the timing of exposure in relation to health effects. The precautionary principle becomes highly important in protecting children. The potentially high and unregulated exposures of children to these chemicals, many of which persist in the environment, increase the vulnerability of children in all parts of the world.

Arsenic

Acute poisoning caused by arsenic is a critical and widespread problem, especially in Bangladesh and parts of India, because of naturally contaminated groundwater accessed by tube wells, and is a sporadic problem elsewhere. The risks of cancer, skin disease, and neurotoxicity associated with arsenic are well known. Arsenic has been associated with an increased prevalence of malnutrition in Bangladeshi children, suggesting a "wasting" effect in the presence of nutritional deficiency, independent of helminth load [24]. This problem has been approached by marking individual wells to inform the public which are safe for use as drinking water and which should be reserved for only nonconsumptive uses. The conventional approach to individual treatment, chelation, is not satisfactory at low levels of exposure and for treating large populations.

Arsenic has a broader spectrum of toxicity, however, than these high-level effects. Recent studies [18] suggest that arsenic is also a risk factor, along with lead, mercury, and deficiency in omega-3 fatty acid intake, for reduced measurable intelligence and academic performance. This observation places another independent variable in the neurodevelopmental risk equation and may argue for review of the current risk assessment for arsenic-associated disease, which is driven by cancer risk [25].

Population risks to which children are uniquely vulnerable

Climate change

Global climate change affects all people. The unique vulnerability of children to its effects arises from the social realities of their predicament: dependency on adults for shelter, food, clean water, and health care [26].

Chaotic weather conditions, which give rise to more frequent and intense weather events, create an increasing responsibility for protecting children from such events as storms, heat waves, and cold snaps. Recent events that have tested emergency preparedness, such as Hurricane Katrina in 2005, the Aceh tsunami in 2004, and several earthquakes affecting Iran, Pakistan, and Indonesia, underscore the need for effective disaster preparedness to protect the lives of children. Sea-level rise, in coastal regions, creates a flood risk. Emergencies on this scale also disrupt families, create great social insecurity, add to poverty, and interfere with schooling and normal

childhood. They demand of the child resilience they should not be expected
to have before adulthood.

The rise in sea level, salt-water intrusion into coastal aquifers, increasing
aridity caused by warming, and stress on oceans (possibly in combination
with overfishing) may result in complex, disruptive effects mediated by increasing costs for water and food, poverty, and social dislocation. These effects are difficult to predict because they act through complicated social
mechanisms and their outcomes, such as substance abuse, physical abuse,
and family insecurity, also have many other causes and influences.

Child malnutrition is already a major cause or contributor to illness in
children worldwide, particularly in less-industrialized society. Climate
change further impacts food availability. The nutritional content of food
produced may be decreased. Increased evaporation in warming climates
may reduce soil moisture and affect agricultural production. Flooding
may decrease crop growth in other settings.

Biologic changes related to climate change include changes in the distribution of infectious disease (both pathogens and vectors) and allergens, in
particular ragweed [27]. These changes in the underlying epidemiology of
disease affect children and adults.

Sanitation

Sanitation is a broad category of hazard control efforts that, essentially,
imply protection of human beings from their own waste and control of conditions that increase the risk of disease from "natural" environmental hazards in human communities. The single most important topic in sanitation,
clean water, is discussed next. Other basic issues in sanitation include the
safe disposal of sewage, the prevention of food-borne illness, and the prevention of breeding grounds for vectors of infectious disease.

Sewage disposal is highly variable around the world. Approximately 2.4
billion people in the world do not have access to a proper toilet [1]. Hand
washing is far from universal in developed countries, let alone in developing
countries and in places where water is in short supply. The potential for
fecal-oral contamination is a constant, worldwide problem. The outcome,
in most cases, is diarrhea. In an adult, diarrhea can be debilitating but unless
there is malnutrition or concomitant illness or the cause of the diarrhea is
cholera, it is usually a transient and self-limited problem. Children, however,
are much more susceptible to dehydration. For infants, acute dehydration
may be fatal. Oral rehydration therapy has been very successful in rescuing
children from life-threatening diarrhea, but an outbreak or case that requires it is an indication that prevention has failed.

Food-borne illness is also usually a problem of fecal-oral contamination,
although food can also be contaminated by nonfecal pathogens and by
chemicals. Contamination by night soil (human feces) used for fertilizer,
sewerage water for irrigation, and during food processing can occur but

the most common cause of food contamination is failure to wash hands after a bowel movement. Food can also be contaminated by improper storage and processing methods, particularly if proper attention is not paid to preparation temperature; refrigeration; using separate cutting boards (to prevent cross-contamination, especially from salmonella from raw chicken); and regular washing of surfaces with soap and clean water. Restaurant and food service inspections are conducted by public health agencies for commercial preparation of food. Food preparation at home for family consumption, however, is unregulated everywhere. The total burden of food-borne illness is not known.

Reducing breeding grounds for vectors is critical to the control of infectious diseases, such as malaria. The toll taken by malaria and other parasites on children is vast in regions where these disorders are endemic. In addition to fatalities and the burden of morbidity, chronic disease renders children more susceptible to the effects of diseases of other causes.

Sanitation is, unfortunately, a low priority for most local governments. Investment is not associated with new industry or many jobs. It is critical to the health, productivity, and sustainability of society, however, and the consequences of failure to provide basic sanitation fall most heavily on children.

Safe drinking water

Safe drinking water is the most basic public health need. It has also been the most difficult to provide to the world's population. Protection of the drinking water supply requires isolation of the source (which may be surface water or a well) from potential contamination; treatment (filtration and disinfection); and secure distribution. At any step along the way, contamination of water may occur and threaten human health. Gross contamination of the water source can overwhelm and degrade the water purification system. Filtration, which removes a large fraction of microbial contamination but not viruses, is a necessary step and essential for removal of many disinfection-resistant parasites. Disinfection, which can take many forms, actively kills pathogens, including viruses. If the distribution system leaks and has low pressure (allowing water surrounding the pipes to enter), however, the water can easily be recontaminated. This is why chlorine has been the preferred disinfection agent for many years, despite its role in the formation of halomethanes (halogenated organic compounds associated with cancer risk and now regulated by the US Environmental Protection Agency). Chlorine continues to act downstream as potable water flows through the pipe, whereas other system-level disinfection agents only work in one place and leave the water downstream unprotected.

Ensuring these minimum, essential steps in the drinking water supply requires regular maintenance and investment. Although not technically complicated, a community-level drinking water system cannot run itself after it is built. There must be some continuity in responsibility for it, repair of pipes, and regular purchase of disinfectant. In many developing societies, this maintenance cannot be ensured. For example, in several cities of Zambia, economic reversals in the copper industry resulted in large-scale unemployment. Without income to pay taxes, maintenance of the water supply system broke down. The result was widespread outbreaks of diarrhea and several fatal outbreaks of cholera, where in the past these had been rare.

Food safety

The safety of food is taken for granted. The communication of food safety messages for consumer protection further increases the perception of that safety. Consumers infrequently consider the risk of food-borne infection or the potential magnitude of risk. As a result, food safety may not be traditionally thought of as an environmental risk of great concern in developed countries. Worldwide, however, food safety remains a larger threat. Food-borne pathogens may cause up to 70% of diarrheal illness and a related 3 million deaths in children under the age of 5 in developing countries [28]. Many potentially food-borne illnesses are reportable in some industrialized countries, resulting in a rapid investigation and containment of the causative problem. Reporting is less prevalent, however, in other places.

Food safety presents a challenge to industrialized and developing countries alike. Large numbers of at-risk infants and children may be disproportionately affected because they are already nutritionally or immunologically compromised, subclinically or overtly. National strategies for food protection and safety, through regulation, growing and handling processes, distribution, and consumer education, could impact positively on food safety of these children.

Food-borne disease may be caused by infectious agents and by a range of chemicals. Infectious transmission of clinical illness is well known, although levels of concern may vary with the setting and circumstances.

Particular food-transmitted hazards may include protozoa, such as *Toxoplasma gondii* (and subsequent congenital toxoplasmosis), and *Giardia lamblia* can be widespread [29]. Bacteria can include listeria, salmonella, *Escherichia coli* 0157:H7, *Clostridium botulinum*, *Vibrio cholera*, *Clostridium perfringens*, shigella, campylobacter, and *Staphylococcus aureus*.

Transmission of the HIV virus is greater in the breast-fed offspring of HIV-infected women than in women who formula feed their infants or use other breast milk substitutes [30]. The availability and cost of such substitutes, however, can be prohibitive in many settings. The existence and national support of comprehensive policies are necessary to improve local education and subsequent reduction in transmission rates of HIV.

Chemical exposures, caused by inadequate protection of the food source, may put large segments of the society at risk for toxic ingestions and short- or longer-term impacts of these exposures. In addition, the risk of chemical contaminants in food sources is magnified by the likelihood of unsafe use of chemicals, increased pollution, and a lack of awareness of environmental hazards in developing countries. Food consumption per unit of body weight is greater in children than adults and increases exposure. A child consumes a diet with larger proportions of milk, vegetables and fruits, or juices, if available [31].

Exposure to pesticides, POPs, mercury, lead, nitrate and nitrate ingestion, mycotoxins at high levels, and food additives may be decreased through consumer education, public health programs, legislation, and environmental health infrastructure in the country [32]. Risk reduction strategies in some areas may be effected through the implementation of educational strategies on the most local and level, through culturally sensitive programs.

Air quality

There are three types of air pollution that are recognized to have effects on children's health: (1) ambient air pollution, (2) air toxics, and (3) indoor air pollution.

Ambient (outdoor) air pollution in metropolitan regions throughout the world is a mixture consisting predominantly of oxidizing chemicals, carbon monoxide, and small particles, of which the most toxic fraction is "fine particulate matter," particles arising primarily from the accretion of sulfates and nitrates that are sized on the order of 2.5 μm or less. The predominant source is motor vehicle emissions, modified by chemical reactions involving sunlight, with a smaller contribution from fixed sources, such as power plants, although this varies locally and fixed sources usually play a larger role in cities in developing countries.

Studies on the health effects of ambient air pollution have emphasized a wide variety of potential concerns, including neurodevelopmental effects. The principal effects of ambient air pollution on the health of children recognized to date, however, cluster around the effects on asthma, host defenses and immune effects, reproductive outcomes, and the early development of lung capacity.

Asthma is triggered by several air pollutants individually and in combination, including oxides of nitrogen, ozone, and fine particulate matter [33]. The evidence that ambient air pollution causes asthma in the first place, however, is weak, although it is well established that peaks in air pollution are associated with increased symptoms, medication usage, and emergency room visits among children with asthma. Ozone affects macrophage processing of foreign proteins and may enhance sensitization when an atopic child is exposed to air pollution in the presence of common antigens. There is limited evidence that children in areas with heavy air pollution develop asthma earlier than those where air pollution is less. The cumulative prevalence of asthma among children does not seem to correlate with local air pollution in the community, including ozone. This may be explained if the effect of air pollution is to accelerate the development of allergy and other atopic disorders in the fraction of children in the population with a hereditary predisposition to allergy. This explanation requires further exploration, because it may be fundamental to interpreting the epidemiologic findings.

Host defenses and immune mechanisms seem to be affected by ambient air pollution in complex ways. The attack rate of viral infections is increased with high levels of air pollution, an effect reproducible in the laboratory, and this may mediate some effects of air pollution in childhood [34].

Prenatal exposure to air pollutants, specifically ozone and carbon monoxide, and high levels of fine particulates, have been associated with adverse fetal health and birth outcomes in several studies [35–37].

The early development of lung function is affected by various environmental factors, including exposure to oxides of nitrogen and fine particulate air pollution. The predominant effect may be associated with compromise in host defense, because the effect of viral infection during early childhood on future lung function is well documented [34].

Indoor air pollution poses health risks to children and adults. The routes of exposures differ in developing countries as compared with developed countries and must be considered accordingly. Open fires are frequently used indoors, and increase ambient particulate matter. Cooking and heating may include the use of wood; crop residues; coal; and dung (biomass fuels) [38]. Exposures may be further concentrated as a result of small, dense family living quarters. Health effects in children may include acute lower respiratory tract infections, and severe infant morbidity and mortality [39].

Secondary exposure to arsenic or fluorine may occur as a result of exposure to "dirty coal" burning [40]. Skin, mucocutaneous membrane irritation, and ocular and upper respiratory tract symptoms may result from nitrogen dioxide and sulfur dioxide exposure [41]. Wood smoke particles may cause respiratory tract symptoms and lead to asthma exacerbation.

Such exposures and symptoms can be reduced through educational programs focusing on cooking habits, increased outdoor work, temporary removal of the child from the most concentrated environments, and so forth. Although such efforts may not completely eliminate the problem, they are inexpensive and easy to implement through public health efforts [42].

The effects of environmental tobacco smoke exposure have been well documented, including increased incidence of asthma, pneumonia, and middle ear effusion [43]. A causal relationship of sudden infant death syndrome with environmental tobacco smoke exposure has been reported. Education and public awareness have helped to reduce smoking rates in the United States; similar efforts could be beneficial worldwide.

Indoor carbon monoxide exposure puts children at risk to tobacco smoke, fires, automobile exhausts, and poorly functioning appliances. It has a higher prevalence in poorly ventilated residences.

Volatile organic compounds have a greater concentration indoors than outdoors, and are found in many household materials or furnishings. Studies are ongoing to determine which volatile organic compounds are associated with specific health effects [22]. Formaldehyde can accentuate respiratory disease, such as asthma, particularly in young children who are often situated in a lower breathing level [44].

Many nations are increasingly adopting WHO ambient air quality guidelines. Strategies have not been implemented as effectively in the developing world, however, and exposures to potentially unhealthy levels of pollution in many settings remain high.

Summary

The principal international organizations for the protection of children from environmental hazards are agencies of the United Nations. WHO, an agency of the United Nations [1], compiles authoritative information on threats to children, monitors trends, and provides technical support and encouragement for programs at the national level. WHO works closely with the United Nations Children's Fund, universally known as UNICEF, which has a broader mandate for children's health and welfare. UNICEF has special programs on sanitation and clean water, disease prevention, and emergency response.

There are numerous nongovernmental organizations that support the goals of children's environmental health and elimination of exposure to environmental hazards, but relatively few devoted specifically to children's environmental health. The most extensive is a network of individuals and organizations known as the International Network for Children's Health, Environment and Safety [45]. This group relies on a network of member-correspondents for updated information and welcomes new participants. It is closely aligned with the International Society of Doctors for the Environment.

Because of their predominance in research and demonstration projects, much of the work of US government agencies is influential in other countries. The Environmental Protection Agency Office of Children's Environmental Health, the National Institute of Environmental Health Sciences, and the Centers for Disease Control and Prevention all play some role on the international stage.

What is ahead for children's environmental health? What should take priority? For purposes of global aid, there is no question that clean water is the highest priority. Beyond that goal, however, it is not clear that there is a "one size fits all" rational prioritization of hazards. A simple global agenda is appealing but not very practical. Environmental threats to children do not divide neatly between developed and developing countries, but rather are local and so vary from place to place.

The alternative approach is to concentrate on building the capacity of the public health and medical systems to protect children in every country. This means raising awareness, creating offices for children's health, building the institutions, knitting together the networks, and educating a generation of practitioners and advocates. Single solutions and single-threat approaches may solve one problem at a time but the threats to children's health require commitment and follow-through on many fronts at once.

References

[1] Commission for Economic Cooperation. Children's health and the environment: a first report on available indicators and measures. Geneva: World Health Organization; 2006.
[2] Gordon B, Mackay R, Rehfuess E. Inheriting the world: the atlas of children's health and the environment. Geneva: World Health Organization; 2004.
[3] Berg KK, Zabel EW, Staley PK, et al. Death of a child after ingestion of a metallic charm—Minnesota 2006. MMWR Morb Mortal Wkly Rep 2006;55:340–1.
[4] Patel AB, Williams SV, Frumkin H, et al. Blood lead in children and its determinants in Nagpur, India. Int J Occup Environ Health 2001;7:119–26.
[5] Harper CC, Mathee A, von Schirnding Y, et al. The health impact of environmental pollutants: a special focus on lead exposure in South Africa. Int J Hyg Environ Health 2003;206: 315–22.
[6] Kaiser R, Henderson AK, Daley WR, et al. Blood lead levels of primary school children in Dhaka, Bangladesh. Environ Health Perspect 2001;109:563–6.
[7] Albalak R, Noonan G, Buchanan S, et al. Blood lead levels and risk factors for lead poisoning among children in Jakarta, Indonesia. Sci Total Environ 2003;301:75–85.
[8] Centers for Disease Control and Prevention. Elevated blood lead levels among internationally adopted children—United States, 1998. MMWR Morb Mortal Wkly Rep 2000;49:97–100.
[9] Koller K, Brown T, Spurgeon A, et al. Recent developments in low-level lead exposure and intellectual impairment in children. Environ Health Perspect 2004;112:987–94.
[10] Nriagu JO, Blankson ML, Ocran K. Childhood lead poisoning in Africa: a growing public health problem. Sci Total Environ 1996;181:93–100.
[11] Romieu I, Lacasana M, McConnell R. Lead exposure in Latin America and the Caribbean. Lead research group of the Pan-American Health Organization. Environ Health Perspect 1997;105:398–405.
[12] Fallon PR. Child labour: issues and directions for the World Bank. Washington, DC: World Bank; 1998.
[13] National Institute for Occupational Safety and Health (NIOSH). Child labour research needs. recommendations from the NIOSH child labour working team. Washington, DC: U.S. Department of Health and Human Services, Centers for Disease Control and Prevention; 1997.
[14] Fassa AG. Health benefits of eliminating child labour. Geneva: International Labour Association; 2003.
[15] Fee J. Lessons learned when investigating the worst forms of child labour using the rapid assessment methodology. Geneva: International Labour Organization; 2004.
[16] Cox RD, Kolb JC, Galli RL, et al. Evaluation of potential adverse health effects resulting from chronic domestic exposure to the organophosphate insecticide methyl parathion. Clin Toxicol 2005;43:243–53.
[17] McConnell R, Pacheco F, Wahlberg K, et al. Subclinical health effects of environmental pesticide contamination in a developing country: cholinesterase depression in children. Environ Res 1999;81:87–91.

[18] von Ehrenstein OS, Poddar S, Yuan Y, et al. Children's intellectual function in relation to arsenic exposure. Epidemiology 2007;18:44–51.

[19] Erdal S, Buchanan SN. A quantitative look at fluorosis, fluoride exposure, and intake in children using a health assessment approach. Environ Health Persp 2005;113:111–7.

[20] Khan A, Moola MH, Cleaton-Jones P. Global trends in dental fluorosis from 1980 to 2000: a systematic review. SADJ 2005;60:418–21.

[21] Meenakshi MRC. Fluoride in drinking water and its removal. J Hazard Mater 2006;137: 456–63.

[22] American Academy of Pediatrics (AAP). Committee of environmental health: handbook of pediatric environmental health. 2nd edition. Elk Grove Village (IL): American Academy of Pediatrics (AAP); 2003.

[23] Damstra T. Emerging environmental threats: endocrine-disrupting chemicals. In: Pronczuk-Garbino J, editor. Children's health and the environment: a global perspective. Geneva: World Health Organization; 2005. p. 217–23.

[24] Minamoto K, Mascie-Taylor CG, Moji K, et al. Arsenic-contaminated water and extent of acute childhood malnutrition (wasting) in rural Bangladesh. Environ Sci 2005;12:283–92.

[25] Tsuji JS, Benson R, Schoof RA, et al. Health effect levels for risk assessment of childhood exposure to arsenic. Regul Toxicol Pharmacol 2004;39:99–110.

[26] Canadian Institute of Child Health. Changing habits, changing climate: foundation analysis. Ottawa (Canada): CICH; 2001.

[27] Wayne P, Foster S, Connolly J, et al. Production of allergenic pollen by ragweed (*Ambrosia artemisiifolia* L.) is increased in CO2-enriched atmosphere. Ann Allergy Asthma Immunol 2002;88:279–82.

[28] Kaferstein FK. Food safety: a commonly underestimated public health issue. World Health Stat Q 1997;50:3–4.

[29] Gilbert RE. Epidemiology of infection in pregnant women. In: Petersen E, Amboise-Thomas P, editors. Congenital toxoplasmosis; scientific background, clinical management and control. Paris: Springer-Verlag; 2000. p. 135–6.

[30] De Cock KM, Fowler MG, Mercier E, et al. Prevention of mother-to-child HIV transmission in resource-poor countries-translating research into policy and practice. JAMA 2000; 283:1175–82.

[31] Gitterman BA, Bearer CF. A developmental approach to pediatric environmental health. Pediatr Clin North Am 2001;49:1071–83.

[32] Mahoney DB, Moy GC. Foodborne hazards of particular concern for the young. In: Pronzcuk-Garbino J, editor. Children's health and the environment: a global perspective. Geneva: World Health Organization; 2005. p. 133–52.

[33] Millstein J, Gilliland F, Berhane K, et al. Effects of ambient air pollution on asthma medication use and wheezing among fourth-grade school children from 12 southern California communities enrolled in the Children's Health Study. Arch Environ Health 2004;59:505–14.

[34] Frampton MW, Samet JM, Utell MJ. Environmental factors and atmospheric pollutants. Semin Respir Infect 1991;6:185–93.

[35] Salam MT, Millstein J, Li YF, et al. Birth outcomes and prenatal exposure to ozone, carbon monozide, and particulate matter: results from the Children's Health Study. Environ Health Perspect 2005;11:1638–44.

[36] Maisonet M, Correa A, Misra D, et al. A review of the literature on the effects of ambient air pollution on fetal growth. Environ Res 2004;95:106–15.

[37] Lacasana M, Esplugues A, Ballester F. Exposure to ambient air pollution and prenatal and early childhood health effects. Eur J Epidemiol 2005;20:183–99.

[38] Smith KR. Biomass fuels, air pollution and health: a global review. New York: Plenum Press; 1987.

[39] Ezzati M, Kammen DM. Quantifying the effects of exposure to indoor air pollution from biomass combustion on acute respiratory infections in developing countries. Environ Health Perspect 2001;109:481–9.

[40] Smith KR, Samet JM, Romieu I, et al. Indoor air pollution in developing countries and acute lower respiratory infections in children. Thorax 2000;55:518–32.

[41] Samet JM, Lambert WE, Skipper BJ. Nitrogen dioxide and respiratory illnesses in infants. Am Rev Respir Dis 1993;148:1258–65.

[42] Brims FCA. Air quality, tobacco smoke, urban crowding and day care: modern menaces and their effects on health. Pediatr Infect Dis J 2005;24:S152–6.

[43] American Academy of Pediatrics (AAP). Committee on environmental health. environmental tobacco smoke: a hazard to children. Pediatrics 1997;99:228–32.

[44] Krzyzanowski M, Quackenboss J, Lebowitz MD. Chronic respiratory effects of indoor formaldehyde exposure. Environ Res 1990;52:117–25.

[45] International Network for Children's Health, Environment and Safety. Available at: http://www.inchesnetwork.net/. Accessed February 23, 2007.

PEDIATRIC CLINICS
OF NORTH AMERICA

Pediatr Clin N Am
54 (2007) 351–373

ELSEVIER
SAUNDERS

Safe and Healthy School Environments

Robert J. Geller, MD[a,b,*], I. Leslie Rubin, MD[a,c,d],
Janice T. Nodvin, BA[a,c], W. Gerald Teague, MD[a,b],
Howard Frumkin, MD, DrPH[e]

[a]Emory Southeast Pediatric Environmental Health Specialty Unit,
49 Jesse Hill Jr Drive SE, Atlanta, GA 30303, USA
[b]Emory University, Department of Pediatrics, 49 Jesse Hill Jr Drive SE,
Atlanta, GA 30303, USA
[c]Institute for the Study of Disadvantage and Disability, 776 Windsor
Parkway, Atlanta, GA 30342, USA
[d]Morehouse School of Medicine, Department of Pediatrics,
720 Westview Drive SW, Atlanta, GA 30310, USA
[e]National Center for Environmental Health/Agency for Toxic Substances and Disease
Registry, Centers for Disease Control and Prevention, Mail Stop F29,
4770 Buford Highway, Atlanta, GA 30341, USA

In the United States, more than 56 million students attend 125,000 public and private elementary, middle, and secondary schools [1–3]. Children spend more time in schools than in any place except home. Millions of adults spend their work lives in these same schools.

Schools are unique environments in many ways. There are few other settings where people spend extended periods of time in such close quarters. The average school has an occupant density somewhere between that of prisons and commercial airplanes, much higher than the average workplace. School buildings often are facilities in need of improvement. Research by the US General Accounting Office [4–6] in the mid-1990s and later by the US Department of Education [7] found that one third of schools had buildings requiring extensive repair or replacement, and almost 60% had at least one major feature needing substantial repair, renovation, or replacement. In addition, about half of the schools reported at least one unsatisfactory environmental condition, such as poor ventilation,

This article is based in part on Frumkin H, Geller RJ, Rubin IL, and Nodvin J, editors. Safe and Healthy School Environments. New York: Oxford University Press; 2006.

* Corresponding author. Emory Southeast Pediatric Environmental Health Specialty Unit, 49 Jesse Hill Jr Drive SE, Atlanta, GA 30303.

E-mail addresses: rgeller@georgiapoisoncenter.org; robert_geller@oz.ped.emory.edu (R.J. Geller).

inadequate heating or lighting, or insufficient physical security. There were schools in warm climates without working air conditioning, schools in cold climates without adequate heat, and schools across the country without good lighting. There were overcrowded schools, noisy schools, and schools with blatant safety hazards. There were exposures to asbestos, lead, petroleum products in underground storage tanks, and radon. In most cases, the problems were not isolated; a school with one problem usually had multiple problems. A recent review of air quality in schools revealed that problems with inadequate ventilation, excessive levels of carbon dioxide, volatile organic compounds, bioaerosols, bacteria, dust mites, and animal allergens were common [8].

Teachers, administrators, and other school staff are protected by a patchwork of Federal, state and local occupational safety regulations, although their scope is narrow in many areas. Staff may be able to request reassignment out of problem areas and obtain support from a union or peers, but students lack such avenues. Unsatisfactory school environmental conditions such as those mentioned previously pose short-term and long-term threats to children's health and productivity [9–11] and may translate into health care costs as well.

The school environment, in the authors' view, is the total experience that surrounds students and the adults who work with them, in the classroom and also on the playing fields and other extracurricular school-related activities, in the cafeteria, and on the way to and from school. It includes obvious environmental factors such as noise, light, and air quality, as well as less obvious factors such as the food choices available to students at school, crime in the vicinity of the school, and the safety of the students' routes between home and school [12,13]. The school environment needs to serve all students at the facility, including those who have disabilities. Applying the principles of environmental health to schools can provide otherwise unavailable opportunities for improving the school setting [9,14,15].

This article focuses on several environmental concerns at school: emergency preparedness, the physical environment of the school, safety and hazard avoidance both on playgrounds and sports fields and within the school, nutrition at school, and concerns about transportation to and from school. Environmental approaches to safe and healthy schools need to be complemented by behavioral approaches to maximize the injury-prevention benefits. Such behavioral interventions include appropriate supervision by properly qualified adults in settings such as pools, playgrounds, and sporting venues. Behavioral approaches to injury prevention have been reviewed extensively elsewhere [16–19]. Also not addressed further here are concerns about asthma at school, air quality inside and outside the school, mold at school, accommodating the needs of diverse individuals who have a range of abilities all are important topics that are covered elsewhere in this issue and others. The broad range of this article precludes comprehensive coverage of any single topic, although each is covered more extensively elsewhere [20].

The article presents several ways in which pediatricians can be effective advocates and partners to promote improvements in the school settings while still working in the context of constrained resources. The importance of a team approach to safe and healthy school environments is emphasized. Schools are complex social systems with many stakeholders. Administrators, parents, staff, neighbors, students, local health care providers, and others need to work together. No school has all the resources it needs to pay its teachers and staff, educate its children, and improve its physical plant, but some issues can be addressed at little expense by changes in policy and practice [21]. If a school cannot afford a deluxe approach, optimizing every aspect of the school environment, a more selective approach may be necessary. Schools can set priorities by systematically addressing needs and opportunities. Excellent tools to guide an assessment are readily available on the Internet (including the recently introduced US Environment Protection Agency [EPA] [22] Healthy School Environmental Assessment Tool program and the Healthy Schools Network [www.healthyschools.org]) and in print [20].

Physical environment of the school

Schools can be designed to be high-performance schools, blending health, performance, environmental, and economic considerations. In this context, high-performance schools are those built to maximize function and minimize environmental impact. This approach is most practical when a new building is constructed or when additions to existing buildings are under way. In considering school design, the initial investment in a high-performance school may seem prohibitively expensive, but a longer-term view may show that the added cost can pay for itself in a few years. "Green" buildings designed to minimize energy use are expensive initially but may provide rapid payback in light of current energy costs. The frugal decision at times may call for spending *more* money. In a recent study of "green" schools, annual financial benefits exceed the costs of building "green" by more than 15-fold; of these benefits, about 25% represents reduced energy costs, and more than 50% represents increased future earnings for students related to their improved academic performance [23]. Even existing facilities can have their physical environment improved in a stepwise fashion when the need to do so is recognized and made a priority.

School site selection

The choice of the site for a new school impacts the school in multiple ways. The siting of new school buildings all too often is based on land availability, often at the perimeter of the area to be served or on land available inexpensively. Such school placement unfortunately often precludes walking and bicycling to and from school for many children. Consideration should be given to easy accessibility to the community when siting new school buildings. Placing a school adjacent to major highways, however, increases the exposure of school occupants to traffic exhaust, recognized as an airway irritant that likely increases asthma symptoms and related respiratory complaints [24,25].

Concern may arise about contamination from landfills when schools are built in close proximity to them. Sanitary landfills near the school may create unpleasant odors, because gases, usually methane and hydrogen sulfide, may be emitted from the landfill as its contents decompose. Methane is not toxic itself but may displace oxygen if it accumulates in an enclosed space. Hydrogen sulfide, with its characteristic rotten-egg smell, may displace oxygen and also interfere with the body's ability to use oxygen. Because air-flow patterns fluctuate during the day and from day to day based on wind speed, wind direction, and weather, the air should be monitored either continuously for several days or at various times of the day during differing weather conditions when exposure to landfill emissions is of concern [16,26–28].

Schools built on top of old landfills may pose particular concerns about contamination of groundwater or well water (with potential infiltration into underground aquifers used to supply water to the community). A pilot study of schools built on former landfills or other previously contaminated sites found no evidence of contamination of the school environment itself [29]. In an initial analysis using 1999 school data, 438 schools were found to have been built on or within 1 mile of 61 contaminated sites (National Priority List, or NPL, sites) in 16 different communities studied by the EPA. One hundred thirty-eight of these schools (with a total enrollment of more than 92,000 students) had been built directly on the contaminated NPL site. Seventy-six percent of these schools were built above contaminated groundwater plumes. Because of remediation efforts, none of the schools above the plumes are exposed currently to contaminated groundwater. An additional 189,366 children attended schools within 1 mile of an NPL site [29].

Safety and hazard avoidance

Injury prevention, by eliminating or reducing exposure to hazards and the probability of injuries from them, is a key goal for schools. Preventing injuries involves striving for optimal balance between minimizing risk and maximizing student involvement in classroom activities. Safety requires the creation of a conducive environment through facility design, supportive policy, and adherence to safe practices. Teachers, staff, and students all play important roles [30].

Issues to consider are the major safety and health hazards present in the school, the options for addressing each hazard, the associated costs, and the degree of benefit that can be expected from the intervention. Hazards may be present at any point in the school but are more likely to exist at some sites than others. Classroom design should anticipate and support the intended use of the space, including rooms for science laboratories, creative arts, and vocational arts/technical skills. Settings where potentially hazardous equipment is used or stored (including shop classes, theater classes producing scenery or using special effects, and science laboratories), playgrounds, athletic venues, and areas under renovation or immediately adjoining them deserve particular scrutiny. Injury risk also may be greater during specific weather conditions (eg, icy or rainy conditions). Policy and practice should anticipate these risks and establish strategies to address them [30]. These potentially hazardous sites are now considered in more detail.

Class settings

Shop classes and similar specialty classes should be evaluated to assure that equipment is in good repair and regularly maintained and that the use of appropriate safety devices is required. Goggles can be designed to be chemically protective, impact-protective, or both. Even eyewear designed to be generally chemically protective will not protect against all chemical hazards, and these limitations should be known and compared against the materials in use. Similarly, chemically protective gloves are designed to protect only against specific types of chemical hazards. Where heat is being generated, in settings such as culinary classes or kiln firing, protective attire must protect against the thermal injury; where welding is occurring, specific attire to protect the user and other occupants of the area must be required.

Chemical exposures

Children may be more susceptible than adults to injury from toxic exposures. They are in the process of maturation and have higher metabolic demands as well as higher minute ventilation in early childhood [31].

Outside the school, some materials, including wood and roofing products treated with copper-chromate-arsenate, pose a hazard for toxic exposure. Exposure in the school building from lead and asbestos (in insulation or flooring) is a concern, especially during periods of substantial renovation.

Exposure risks during renovations

Teaching activities should not be held in an area undergoing substantial renovation (eg, removal of walls, stripping of paint or finishes, or replacement of windows), if at all possible. These areas should remain closed until the proper cleaning has been completed. The degree to which the area should be isolated varies according to circumstances and from one phase of construction to another. In this setting, the most likely route of toxicity is through inhalation of dust and particles; the most common health effects are respiratory irritation, development of asthma or airway disease, and worsening of respiratory conditions.

Renovation of older buildings presents risks from asbestos exposure. Until the 1970s, asbestos was used as an insulation material and pipe covering and in concrete flooring. When asbestos materials are intact, they pose no toxic hazard. Once disturbed, however, the fine fibers of asbestos can circulate in the air for long periods of time. Once inhaled, these particles settle in the lungs. Because of the small size of the fibers, the lungs are unable to clear them effectively and instead begin an inflammatory reaction around them. This process can lead to scarring and permanent lung damage. The particles can cause prompt respiratory irritation, but the most serious health effects are delayed, including long-term lung damage and the potential development of cancer. Although these long-term effects are seen primarily in people who have worked with asbestos materials in industry or have been exposed during abatement work, using caution to minimize any exposure during reconstruction and abatement is appropriate.

Asbestos exposure also can occur during excavation activities at sites where the soil contains naturally occurring asbestos [32]. At sites where this or similar conditions exist, appropriate precautions may be necessary to minimize dispersion of asbestos particles.

Asphalt is used to coat roofing materials and road surfaces; because it is hot when applied, burns are a risk. As asphalt cools, it produces a characteristic and offensive odor and can give off toxic fumes containing hydrocarbons, methane, propane, hydrogen sulfide, and carbon monoxide. During ongoing roofing at school, children and staff should be kept away from the areas where there is active use of asphalt. Generally these construction activities occur outside, where ample fresh air provides natural ventilation. Building air intakes located near asphalt activities can suck the odor and fumes into a building, however [33–35]. Fumes from cooling asphalt may result in shortness of breathing, dizziness, or lightheadedness, as well as nausea, from the hydrocarbons and carbon monoxide. Hydrogen sulfide has a strong odor and most commonly causes irritation to the eyes, nose, and throat as well as difficulty breathing. People who exhibit symptoms after exposure to cooling asphalt should be removed from the area immediately into fresh air. Anyone who faints or has persistent symptoms should be evaluated by medical personnel.

Chemical exposures outdoors and indoors

Concerns may occur regarding contamination of nearby groundwater and soil from particles of rooftop material or substances from the environment that have accumulated on the roof. To date, there are no data proving a harmful effect on humans from rooftop runoff. Roofing materials include galvanized metals or asphalt shingles, typically containing heavy metals such as zinc and cadmium. Other metals often are present also but in much smaller amounts. In rural schools using well water as drinking water, however, groundwater and well water should be tested periodically to minimize risk [36,37].

Within the school, a hazard for lead poisoning may exist. Common sources include old paint containing lead and plumbing leaching lead into the water. The hazards of lead from old paint are well known to most pediatricians, but the risk of lead contamination of drinking water may be less familiar. The EPA recommends that water sampled from drinking faucets contain less than 20 ppb of lead [38]. Surveys of schools in several communities in Maryland and Pennsylvania found faucets exceeding this standard in more than 20% of schools tested [38].

In the classroom, toxic exposure can result from arts and crafts supplies or theater makeup, sets, and special-effects materials. Students and teachers in shop class are at risk for exposure from solvents and glue; paints, varnishes, and other finishes; metal reactions; and wood by-products. Office equipment and supplies can cause respiratory and skin irritation in sensitive people. When new, pressed-wood products (such as used in some furniture and some modular buildings) often emit formaldehyde fumes, a known airway irritant.

Arts and crafts supplies should be selected by considering their hazards as well as their features. The Art and Creative Materials Institute has developed labels for art supplies that designate their level of toxicity [39]. The CP seal and the AP seal indicate that a product is nontoxic even if ingested. The CL seal indicates that a product contains toxic ingredients. Products labeled with the CL seal can be used safely, if used with caution. The HL seal indicates that a product contains one or more toxic components in sufficient quantities to have an immediate or long-term effect on health. Products with CL seals (eg, rubber cement containing n-hexane) should be used only by people who can read, understand, and follow the directions for safe use. Such products should be avoided when working with young children. If there is doubt about the potential toxicity of a product, the product's Materials Safety Data Sheet (MSDS) should be obtained and reviewed with an occupational safety expert, certified industrial hygienist, or similarly knowledgeable individual before the product is purchased or used.

Careful selection of chemicals to be used within the school can minimize the risk of toxicity. The usefulness and safety of chemicals used in the processes of cleaning, maintenance, and renovation and in the classrooms themselves should be evaluated. The MSDS information about the potential hazards and storage needs of each chemical should be reviewed before the chemical is purchased . If the chemical is purchased after this initial review, the MSDS should be kept at the school in a readily accessible location.

A complete manifest of all chemicals used within the school should be developed and updated at least annually. All chemicals should be stored safely, in keeping with local and Federal standards, and access to them should be restricted to qualified staff [31].

Crowding

If the school facility feels crowded subjectively, the performance and well-being of students, teachers, and other school staff will be affected adversely. Performance is affected by crowding both within a specific classroom and within the school overall [40].

Two concepts help explain the experience of crowding: privacy and overstimulation. High density may result in feelings of being crowded because in this setting people have a difficult time achieving privacy. Privacy is the perceived ability to control interactions with others, not just the ability to be alone. Privacy may be obtained by getting away from other people, but it also can be achieved by limiting the number of other people with whom one has to interact.

Overstimulation is another reason that crowding affects school performance. A learning situation requires a high level of sustained attention; in the classroom, children must pay attention for extended periods of time. In addition to the lesson material, other sources of stimulation (eg, bulletin board displays, decorations on classroom walls, other students) are present in the classroom. Further distraction may come from uncontrolled constant interaction with other people, as a result of large group size or high spatial density. Sustained focused learning in a high-density classroom, especially for difficult or complex material, can result in attentional overload or cognitive fatigue. Cognitive fatigue in turn interferes with learning—children no longer are able to attend to the lesson content [41]. Time away from a high-density classroom (eg, for outdoor activities or for a trip to the school library) may help relieve cognitive fatigue. If unable to take such a break, children may just tune out or daydream, at a loss of valuable learning time. Children who have attention-deficit hyperactivity disorder or autism-spectrum conditions are particularly vulnerable to crowding and overstimulation; any change in a child's performance or behavior should be examined in this context.

Another possible outcome, particularly in children from crowded homes, is the development of motivational problems, also called "learned helplessness" [42]. When confronted with too much stimulation, such as the constant presence of other people with whom interaction is occurring, affected children no longer are motivated to pay attention or complete a task. This problem is more likely to happen when a task is complex or difficult. When placed in a situation of sustained crowding, these children learn to be helpless; they simply give up when things get difficult.

School size, class size, and furniture arrangements can be modified to alleviate crowded conditions. Each crowded setting should be addressed individually, by modification of one or more of these factors.

Recently, some communities have experienced rapid population movement into areas that have become attractive quickly, resulting in schools that suddenly have a much higher number of students than the existing school building can accommodate. Often, these schools must use temporary facilities, such as portable buildings or trailers. The consequences of this arrangement on the students and the teachers who must spend their days in the trailers, as well as on the impact on the school and on the neighborhood, has yet to be evaluated adequately.

Lighting

Whether the school is heavily occupied or not, lighting is a key feature of the school environment. Appropriate lighting requires adequate brightness as well as even, glare-free lighting of a balanced spectrum. Good lighting can improve health and learning as well as enhance safety, reduce vandalism, and help students connect visually to their environment, at the same time reducing energy expenditures.

A comprehensive approach to optimal lighting includes using daylight and providing outdoor views in all classrooms and work areas, combining daylight and electric lighting to prevent shadows and areas of poor illumination during cloudy days or during darkness, and the addition of flexible lighting controls [43]. A direct correlation between student learning and lighting quality has been demonstrated in a study of three school districts. Students with more daylight in their classrooms progressed more than 20% faster in math and reading skills than their counterparts in classrooms without daylight [44].

Just why students perform better in spaces that provide daylight is unclear. The quality of lighting affects the ability to see the information presented and to sort through complex tasks more quickly, and daylight's potential for higher quality and quantity of light may give students the advantage of clear and precise sight. Lighting also affects moods and general health, and the demonstrated changes in performance may be explained, at least in part, by improvements in the health or mood of students, teachers, or both. Prolonged periods of low light levels (such as those occurring at high latitudes in winter) can cause seasonal depression and reduced performance (seasonal affective disorder) for some people [45]. Persons who have mild seasonal affective disorder should be encouraged to spend time in a brightly lit outdoor space every day.

Temperature and humidity

School buildings in the United States and other technologically developed countries have heating and air-conditioning systems designed to maintain a comfortable environment for the building occupants. People's perceptions of thermal comfort are affected principally by three environmental parameters: temperature, humidity, and air movement. Physical activity and clothing, interacting with the use of the space, also play an important role. For example, the ideal temperature for classrooms (21°–23°C; 69.8°–73.4°F) is higher than for gymnasiums because of the lower level of exercise usually occurring in the classroom and the different clothing worn by the occupants within.

Excessively warm or cold school buildings adversely affect attentiveness, performance, and indoor air quality overall [46,47]. The term "sick building syndrome" has been used to describe a set of symptoms common among office workers in buildings with indoor air problems. The main components of sick building syndrome generally are regarded as nasal, eye, and mucous membrane symptoms, lethargy, dry skin, and headaches. The occurrence of symptoms related to sick building syndrome is reduced at optimal indoor temperature and relative humidity.

Humidity can be problematic both when it is too low and when it is too high; an optimal value is probably 40% to 60% relative humidity. Humidifying excessively dry air seems to decrease the incidence of upper respiratory infections [46], but excessive humidity promotes the growth of mold [48] and the persistence of both cockroach and dust mite allergens.

Noise

Excessive noise within the school setting, whether arriving from outside the building or from other points within the building, has been shown to affect adversely student learning and staff productivity and well-being. In a school setting, noise can be considered as any unwanted sound that interferes with classroom communication and is both disturbing and detrimental to the learning process [49].

Both acute and chronic noisy conditions influence learning [49]. Noise adversely impacts the ability of teachers and students to communicate, as well as students' attention, memory, and thus motivation and academic achievement. The most consistent finding is that the effects of chronic noise on learning are most pronounced when a task or activity is difficult or complex or when greater concentration is needed. Because of their difficulty in understanding and processing information, children who have attention difficulties (eg, attention-deficit hyperactivity disorder), learning disabilities, developmental disabilities including sensory impairments (hearing or visual), conditions along the autism spectrum, or intellectual disabilities may require settings with less background noise to focus on their task.

Health issues related to classroom noise include stress and increased blood pressure and heart rates in children—conditions that may persist into adulthood. Teachers also can experience mental and voice fatigue [49,50].

Noise is more problematic in classrooms than in other spaces such as gymnasiums. External conditions such as low-flying aircraft overhead, a heavily traveled street, or nearby trains can contribute to a noisy classroom. Classroom noise can be generated by lighting, mechanical ventilation systems, and heating and cooling systems. Classroom activities and sounds from adjacent spaces such as the corridor and music practice rooms also can create problems with noise.

Most efforts to reduce noise are directed at the classroom and at appropriate selection of room adjacencies and scheduling of classroom activities within the building. Careful school planning and design of new buildings and thoughtful modification of existing sites can alleviate noisy conditions in the school. Appropriate noise studies (including reverberation time, signal/noise ratio, and ambient noise level) in classrooms, corridors, cafeterias, music spaces, and other important areas should be obtained to guide interventions.

Creating an optimal acoustical environment for learning requires anticipating likely sources of noise and planning ways to minimize those sources. Classrooms will require mechanical systems for air circulation and thermal comfort. Lighting systems and instructional equipment such as computers and projectors contribute to ambient noise. Activities within the space generate noise. Lecture spaces require acoustical properties different from those needed in classrooms, where multiple simultaneous conversations occur.

Learning spaces requiring quiet must be located away from traditionally noisy areas such as cafeterias and athletic areas. Some spaces—music practice and athletic areas, for example—must be isolated to protect the rest of the school from the noise generated there. Appropriately designed walls, floors, ceilings, and roofs can reduce noise transmission to adjacent spaces significantly. In existing schools, walls, floors, and ceilings may require acoustical treatment to reduce noise levels. Some teachers use carpeting and other soft, sound-absorbent material on floors and walls to create better acoustical conditions, but carpeting alone usually does not provide enough sound absorption to solve classroom noise problems [43]. Full-height walls reduce noise transmission. Appropriate doors, windows, and skylights can diminish noise transmission from within the school and from external sources of noise [43].

Nutrition at school

Food service within the school occurs throughout the day, both at meal times and between meals (often through automated vending equipment). Appropriate selection of foods and their attractive presentation can influence school performance as well as help develop habits to address the current national epidemic of obesity [51,52]. Foods must be stored and preserved safely to minimize the risk of food-transmitted illness [10,53]. Pediatricians can be advocates for reducing the availability of foods and drinks of low nutritional value within the school.

Pest control at school

In the past pest control was synonymous with routine spraying of pesticides. Major disadvantages of this approach have been recognized, both in its expense and in its potential exposure to hazardous chemicals. Integrated pest management (IPM), based on information on the life cycles of pests, how they interact with the environment, and what they need to survive, is a preferred approach. IPM emphasizes nonchemical means of control, such as creating inhospitable environments, removing sources of food, blocking entry into buildings, and placing traps.

Pesticides also are used in IPM programs but in a judicious, targeted way. If the level of pests exceeds that acceptable to the school personnel, the least toxic appropriate pesticides should be used in the smallest application suitable for controlling the problem. Baits and gels in schools are almost always preferred to other pesticide application methods because their highly specific application minimizes human exposure [54,55].

Playgrounds

Playgrounds and other play spaces present a paradox. They need to stimulate children's imaginations and offer opportunities to explore, create, expend energy, and take risks—all normal parts of growing up. Playgrounds also need to be safe. Playground injuries are a leading cause of injury to elementary and junior high students, ages 5–14 years, while at school [56]. Based on published studies, the US Office of Technology Assessment concluded that the most common settings for unintentional school injuries are playgrounds, gymnasiums, and athletic fields [57]. Injuries associated with playgrounds are the most prevalent and account for 30% to 45% of unintentional school injuries.

Tinsworth and McDonald [58] analyzed the US Consumer Product Safety Commission (CPSC) data files regarding playground equipment related to 147 deaths between 1990 and 2000. At public playgrounds, including both schools and parks, about four deaths per year were reported over the 10-year period. The three most common causes of death were strangulation (54%), falls to nonresilient surfaces such as asphalt (21%), and equipment tip-over or collapse (16%). Strangulation usually results from entangled clothing or cords caught on equipment, most often slides. Thus, efforts at reducing playground deaths should emphasize three areas: appropriate clothing without protruding cords, adherence to the CPSC guidelines regarding playground equipment and the surfaces below the equipment, and good maintenance of equipment [56].

Playground injuries with nonfatal outcomes occur much more often. An estimated 205,850 playground equipment–related injuries were treated in hospital emergency rooms in the United States during a 12-month period from November 1998 to October 1999, according to data gathered through the National Electronic Injury Surveillance System [58]. Of these, 70,218 (45%) were associated with playground equipment in schools. In school settings, 28% of play-equipment injuries also involved other children.

Playground injuries were categorized as fractures (39%), lacerations (22%), contusions and abrasions (20%), and strains and sprains (11%). Almost 80% of fractures involved the elbow, lower arm, or wrist. Body areas most frequently affected in school-aged children were the arm and hand (43%) and head and face (34%). About 15% of injuries to the face and head were diagnosed as concussions, internal injuries, and fractures.

Falls were involved in 79% of these public playground-equipment injuries in schools and other settings. Only 3% of all playground injuries required hospitalization; all were the result of falls. These data demonstrate that falls present the greatest risk to children using playground equipment and account for a disproportionately large percentage of severe injuries.

The death of a child is always a tragedy, but the average of four playground-equipment deaths each year is much lower than the estimated 37 killed by another vehicle while waiting for school buses, the 20 deaths related to sports injury each year, or the 44 school homicides annually [57].

Moore [56] discusses how several authorities have suggested that the balance of safety and risk has tipped too far toward safety. They cite two reasons: the constraints imposed by the Americans with Disabilities Act Guidelines for Play Areas [59] and the focus on legal liability. One unintended consequence of the Americans with Disabilities Act may be that the change in play environments has removed appropriate levels of challenge for the large majority of children who are able-bodied. Such risk aversion can reduce the play value of playgrounds. A more balanced approach would reconcile the value of play in healthy child development with choice of environmental accessibility and appropriate emphasis on safety.

The pediatric health care provider can be an effective advocate for addressing these competing priorities. Thoughtful and creative playground design and careful maintenance of play equipment and the surrounding cushioning surfaces are essential components of promoting outdoor play.

Sports venues

The inherent risks in outdoor sports participation can be mitigated by careful design and maintenance of playing fields, adequate lighting, and protective fencing. Indoor sports injuries can result from inappropriate use of space or inadequate equipment. Soccer, football, baseball, basketball, and gymnastics all present specific safety issues for participants and spectators.

Sports injuries occur during organized sports and during unsupervised sporting activities. Sixty-two percent of injuries occurring during organized sports happen during practice [60]. Although baseball causes fewer injuries than bicycling, basketball, or football, it has the highest fatality rate among sports for children ages 5–14 years [60]. The CPSC analyzed the 88 reports it received of baseball-related deaths of children between 1973 and 1995. It found that 68 of the deaths were caused by ball impact, and 13 were caused by bat impact. Of the 68 ball-impact deaths, 38 resulted from blows to the chest; 21 deaths were caused by a ball hitting a player's head [61].

Field sports share several common safety precautions. Fields should be assessed, before each use, for hazards that may have developed. Any accumulated debris should be removed before the field is used. If the debris cannot be removed and the hazards addressed before use, the field should not be used. Field equipment, including soccer and football goals, must be attached securely and padded appropriately. Fencing around the field should be well secured and in good repair, without sharp edges.

Indoor sports also share common safety considerations. The site should be in good repair, without hazard of falling debris or floor defects. The boundaries around the sports area should be large enough to allow athletes to come to a safe stop after going out of bounds, to reduce the risk of knee or ankle injuries from sudden deceleration. Gymnastics and cheerleading areas should have appropriately padded surfaces. Water fountains should be situated to minimize the risk of athletes slipping on spilled water.

Injuries during baseball, football, and soccer can be minimized by using the suggestions in Box 1 [62]. The relationship between players heading the ball and brain damage in soccer players is complex. Studies of soccer head injuries show that the ball was involved in less than 25% of concussions, and few, if any, concussions occurred during uninterrupted purposeful heading. The average number of headings per game was not a significant risk factor for concussions. The possibility of long-term effects from heading remains controversial [63]. Discouraging younger players from heading the ball is a prudent practice until better information is available to resolve this issue.

Drowning is another all-too-frequent cause of an emergency department visit and is often fatal. Schools should model pool safety and safe swimming practices for students and staff alike. Appropriate safety guidelines at poolside include [62]

- The pool should be locked when not in use to avoid unauthorized usage.
- A pool maintenance company or a trained school employee should provide daily chemical analysis of the water and maintain a log of results.
- Deep areas should be at least 10 feet deep to allow diving, and the slope of the pool floor should be gradual enough to reduce neck and spine injuries to students diving.
- The depth of the water should be posted around the perimeter of the pool, and "no diving" signs should be posted where appropriate.

Box. 1. Strategies for injury reduction during sports

Baseball

The top of the fence should be padded along the outfield and foul lines.

A 6- to 8-foot warning track of dirt or crushed brick (rather than grass) should be installed between the edges of the field and any fence, so that players chasing a fly ball will be warned that they are nearing the fence.

The dugouts and player bench areas should be fenced to shield them from batted or thrown balls and thrown bats.

The bullpen, or relief pitcher warm-up area, should be fenced and should provide an area for another player to watch for approaching balls and warn the players who are warming up.

Similarly, the "on deck" area (warm-up area for the next batter), if used, should be located beside or behind the dugout to decrease the risk of being struck by a wild pitch, foul ball, or thrown bat.

The bases should be the breakaway type that detach when a player slides into them. These safety-release bases, which leave no holes in the ground or parts of the base sticking up from the ground when the base is released, have been shown to prevent or reduce the severity of the approximately 6600 base-contact sliding injuries to the foot, ankle, and knee occurring annually [61].

Football and soccer

Each drainage grate in the field surface should be marked with visible orange cone.

The corner boundaries should be marked with flexible or collapsible stakes to reduce the risk of injury to players from hitting the boundary marker.

The yard line markers should be made of padded material rather than wood.

Soccer balls should be made of waterproof synthetic material rather than leather, because waterlogged leather balls become heavy and therefore dangerous.

The goalposts for both soccer and football should be padded, and the end zone markers should be made of soft collapsible material or weighted with sand to allow them to stand up. Padding the goalposts will reduce head injuries from direct contact with the goalpost by players not wearing head protection.

Heat- and cold-induced sports illnesses

Heat illness is one of the most common preventable and potentially cat-astrophic problems in sports [62]. Although it accounts for only 2 to 5 deaths each year among young athletes, less severe injuries are more com-mon. Thermoregulation is less efficient in young athletes than in adults. Children generate more heat per pound of body weight than adults. They sweat later and less than adults, and they take longer to acclimate to heat and humidity than do adults. These factors place young athletes at increased risk of heat-related illness. Some children (eg, those who are obese or who have cystic fibrosis, poorly controlled asthma, and some other disabilities) are at particularly increased risk of heat stroke.

The severity of heat illness ranges from mild heat cramps to life-threaten-ing heat stroke. Both athletes and coaches must know the early signs of heat illness and know how to prevent it. The best prevention is adequate hydra-tion, both before and during activity.

Thirst is not always a good indicator of fluid needs, so intake of appro-priate amounts of liquid should be encouraged, particularly in hot weather. On the other hand, excess fluid intake can lead to complications (including electrolyte disturbances such as hyponatremia and seizures) as well [64]. The best type of beverage to use in such sports settings has been studied exten-sively; most of these studies suggest that sodium-containing fluids reduce the risk of hyponatremia. Most sports beverages contain only a small amount of sodium, which may be too low to prevent hyponatremia [65–69]. Flavoring the beverage to make it taste better may enhance its acceptance by the ath-letes and improve their fluid balance [70].

To reduce or prevent heat-related illness, young athletes should [62]

- Drink at least enough to quench thirst before the beginning of practice or games.
- Drink appropriate amounts of fluid every 15 to 20 minutes while exer-cising. For most school-aged children, 4 to 12 ounces every 15 to 20 min-utes is probably reasonable.
- Water is usually adequate for activity lasting 1 hour or less, when the fluid intake is less than 32 ounces. If the activity lasts more than 1 hour, a sports drink containing electrolytes (sodium and potassium) and carbohydrates is probably better than either water or a carbonated beverage.
- Traditionally, avoiding salt tablets is recommended because of the dan-ger of excessive sodium intake, although this risk has not been well stud-ied. An important exception to this general rule is a child who has cystic fibrosis.

An athlete suffering a heat-related illness should be removed from activity immediately, allowed to rest in a cool, shaded place, and given fluids to drink. Enhancing cooling (eg, by removing the outer layer of clothes) is often appropriate. Careful monitoring is essential. If the athlete becomes dizzy, disoriented, confused or uunable to drink, ice bags should be applied to the neck, armpits, and groin to speed cooling while emergency medical help is brought to the scene.

At the opposite end of the spectrum, exposure to low temperatures can cause cold-related disorders such as hypothermia and frostbite. Hypothermia can occur with moderate temperatures as high as 65°F, and frostbite can occur when temperatures are 31° and below. Hypothermia can occur, even if the temperature is above freezing, because of sweating and the use of inadequate clothing, especially during rest breaks and windy conditions. Dry clothing should be used to prevent excessive conductive heat loss. As the temperature drops below freezing, the risk of frostbite increases. Covering the exposed skin on the hands and face to minimize exposure helps reduce the chance of frostbite. When the temperature drops to an extremely cold level (compared with the usual climate of the area), outdoor activities should be moved indoors or cancelled.

Transportation

Transportation to and from school represents yet another paradox. On one hand, walking and bicycling offer physical fitness benefits and contribute to decreased motor vehicle mileage, thereby also conferring clean air benefits. These modes of personal transportation are often more hazardous than transport by school bus, however, particularly when schools are not centrally located within the neighborhood they serve or when sidewalks and bicycle paths are not safe and well maintained [12,13]. Implementation of a "Safe Routes to School" program can promote walking and bicycling and also promote improvements in practice and community routes to enhance safety.

The safest means of transportation to and from school remains the traditional school bus [71], particularly if exhaust fumes from the bus are minimized using best practices such as low-sulfur fuels and retrofitting older buses to reduce particle emissions. Transportation by family vehicle or by students driving themselves poses higher risks of injury. Approximately 800 school-age children are killed each year in motor vehicle crashes during school travel hours. These fatalities represent about one in seven of the 5600 child deaths that occur each year on roads in the United States. Only 20 (2%) of these 800 fatalities—5 school bus passengers and 15 pedestrians— are related to school buses. The other 98% of deaths among school-age children involve children in passenger vehicles, walking, bicycling, or riding in buses other than school buses. A majority of the passenger vehicle–related deaths (approximately 450 of the 800 deaths, or 55%) occur when a teenager is driving [67].

Emergency preparedness

Every school should have a general emergency plan. The pediatrician's participation in the development of such a plan allows current medical practice to be incorporated into the plan and allows the local medical community to create its own plans to support the school's occupants if an emergency should develop. Many jurisdictions require schools to have such a plan, but the extent to which the plan is developed may vary from school to school. When schools and communities are prepared to manage emergencies adequately, the extent to which an incident causes harm is minimized [72]. Although less apparent, the process of preparing for emergency incidents often is effective in mitigating the potential for incidents to occur. As a result, emergency preparedness improves the school's ability to respond to an incident and is a preventive strategy as well.

Well-established principles of emergency preparedness can be applied specifically to the school environment. The National Incident Management System, which is required by all recipients of Federal funding, and the similar Incident Command System used by fire and law enforcement authorities throughout the country, are adapted easily for school use. Either system can improve the response capabilities of a school substantially through the effective organization and management of personnel, and provides a framework from which school staff is assigned to work on several defined emergency teams.

At the heart of preparing for school emergencies is the development of an emergency plan to deal with a range of scenarios likely to be encountered within the learning environment. Such situations might include natural disasters, traffic collisions, acts of violence, explosions, fires, and chemical emissions within the adjoining community. Because of regional differences, schools should identify other plausible incidents for inclusion in the emergency plan. For each of the identified events, the emergency plan should define a sequence of initial response actions and procedures.

Within the scope of the overall emergency plan is a first aid/medical segment. The first aid/medical issues that should be addressed include communication procedures, presence of an ambulance and emergency medical help at appropriate times (and how to summon such help if not present, including prewritten instructions on to reach the site to be given to the emergency dispatcher), and proper medical equipment. The emergency plan should be reviewed and updated periodically. It should be rehearsed with all staff. Ideally, all coaches, health care staff, and as many other staff as possible, should be trained in cardiopulmonary resuscitation and the use of an automatic electrical defibrillation device [62].

Specific topics typically addressed in the scope of this segment of the plan also include [72]

- Assigning first aid personnel
- Assessing the available inventory of supplies and equipment

- Setting up first aid treatment areas accessible to emergency vehicles
- Determining the need for and requesting skilled medical assistance
- Overseeing the care, treatment, and assessment of patients
- Keeping the incident commander informed of overall status
- Keeping a log of injured and missing persons, compiled from the reports submitted from the first aid/medical team

During an emergency, the members of the first aid/medical team assess injuries and supply first aid and initial medical treatment as indicated. Specific duties may include setting up areas for triage, first aid, and temporary morgue; keeping accurate records of care given to any injured personnel; and reporting any deaths to the first aid/medical team leader.

The pediatrician may be of particular value in helping refine and update this segment to reflect current understanding of optimal medical management.

Summary

Children spend much of their waking time at school. What they learn at school—both what is taught and what is observed—influences their future, for better or worse. All too often, the school environment adversely affects their educational achievement. Many of the factors in the school environment can be improved with careful planning and allocation of resources. It is important to consider intangible costs and benefits such as community confidence in the school and the value of student and staff comfort. It also is important to analyze limited resources in a long-term context. The pediatrician, as a child advocate, is in an excellent position to influence the allocation of school resources to improve the educational outcome. This article summarizes some of the current understanding gathered from applying an environmental health approach to the school setting and provides a basis for the interested physician and other child advocate to learn more and get involved.

References

[1] Wirt J, Choy S, Rooney P, et al. The condition of education 2006. Washington, DC: US Department of Education, National Center for Education Statistics; 2006. Available at:. http://nces.ed.gov/programs/coe Accessed June 8, 2006.

[2] Broughman SP, Pugh KW. Characteristics of private schools in the United States: results from the 2001-2002 private school Universe Survey. Washington, DC: US Department of Education, National Center for Education Statistics; 2004. Available at: http://nces.ed.gov/pubs2005/2005305.pdf. Accessed June 8, 2006. NCES 2005-305.

[3] Hoffman L. Overview of public elementary and secondary schools and districts: school year 2001–02. Washington, DC: US Department of Education, National Center for Education Statistics; 2003. Available at: http://nces.ed.gov/pubs2003/overview03/index.asp#a. Accessed June 8, 2006. NCES 2003-411.

[4] US General Accounting Office. School facilities: condition of America's schools. Washington, DC: GAO; 1995. Available at: http://www.gao.gov/archive/1995/he95061.pdf. Accessed June 8, 2006. GAO/HEHS-95-61.

[5] US General Accounting Office. School facilities: America's schools report differing conditions. Washington, DC: GAO; 1996. Available at: http://www.gao.gov/archive/1996/he96103.pdf. Accessed June 8, 2006. GAO/HEHS-96-103.

[6] US General Accounting Office. School facilities: profiles of school conditions by state. Washington, DC: GAO; 1996. Available at: http://www.gao.gov/archive/1996/he96148.pdf. Accessed June 8, 2006. GAO/HEHS-96-148.

[7] US Department of Education, National Center for Education Statistics. Condition of America's public school facilities: 1999. Washington, DC: U.S. Department of Education; 2000. Available at: http://nces.ed.gov/surveys/frss/publications/2000032/. Accessed June 8, 2006.

[8] Daisey JM, Angell WJ, Apte MG. Indoor air quality, ventilation and health symptoms in schools: an analysis of existing information. Indoor Air 2003;13:53–64.

[9] Gitterman BA, Bearer CF. A developmental approach to pediatric environmental health. Pediatr Clin North Am 2001;48(5):1071–83.

[10] National Research Council, Committee on Pesticides in the Diets of Infants and Children. Pesticides in the diets of infants and children. Washington, DC: National Academies Press; 1993.

[11] Weiss B. Vulnerability of children and the developing brain to neurotoxic hazards. Environ Health Perspect 2000;108(Suppl 3):375–81.

[12] Braza M, Shoemaker W, Seeley A. Neighborhood design and rates of walking and biking to elementary school in 34 California communities. Am J Health Promot 2004;19(2):128–36.

[13] Dellinger AM, Staunton CE. Barriers to children walking and biking to school—United States, 1999. MMWR Morb Mortal Wkly Rep 2002;51(32):701–4.

[14] Landrigan PJ, Kimmel CA, Correa A, et al. Children's health and the environment: public health issues and challenges for risk assessment. Environ Health Perspect 2004;112(2):257–65.

[15] Lanphear BP, Vorhees CV, Bellinger DC. Protecting children from environmental toxins. PLoS Medicine 2005;2:e61. Available at: http://medicine.plosjournals.org/perlserv/?request=get-document&doi=10.1371/journal.pmed.0020061. Accessed June 8, 2006.

[16] Garcia de Cortazar AL, Lantaron JH, Fernandez OM, et al. Modeling for environmental assessment of municipal solid waste landfills, part 2: biodegradation. Waste Manag Res 2002;20(6):514–28.

[17] Gielen AC, Sleet D. Application of behavior-change theories and methods to injury prevention. Epidemiol Rev 2003;25:65–76.

[18] Liller KD, Sleet DA. Health promotion research approaches to the prevention of injuries and violence. Am J Health Behav 2004;28(Suppl 1):S3–5.

[19] MacKay M, Scanlan A, Olsen L, et al. Looking for the evidence: a systematic review of prevention strategies addressing sport and recreational injury among children and youth. J Sci Med Sport 2004;7:58–73.

[20] Frumkin H, Geller RJ, Rubin IL, et al, editors. Safe and healthy school environments. New York: Oxford University Press; 2006. p. 1–462.

[21] Everett Jones S, Brener ND, McManus T. Prevalence of school policies, programs, and facilities that promote a healthy physical school environment. Am J Public Health 2003;93(9):1570–5.

[22] US Environmental Protection Agency, Office of Children's Health. Healthy school environments assessment tool. 2006. Available at: http://www.epa.gov/schools/healthyseat/index.html. Accessed April 23, 2006.

[23] Kats G, Perlman J, Jamadagni S. National review of green schools: costs, benefits, and implications for Massachusetts. Washington, DC: Capital E; 2005. Available at: http://www.cap-e.com/ewebeditpro/items/O59F7707.pdf. Accessed June 8, 2006.

[24] McConnell R, Berhane K, Yao L, et al. Traffic, susceptibility, and childhood asthma. Environ Health Perspect 2006;114:766–72.

[25] Potera C. The freeway running through the yard: traffic exhaust and asthma in children. Environ Health Perspect 2006;114:A305.
[26] Isidori M, Lavorgna M, Nardelli A, et al. Toxicity identification evaluation of leachates from municipal solid waste landfills: a multispecies approach. Chemosphere 2003;52(1):85–94.
[27] Tarkowski S, Jarup L, Laurent C. Biological monitoring in waste landfills studies. Int J Occup Med Environ Health 2000;13(4):345–60.
[28] Ward ML, Bitton G, Townsend T, et al. Determining toxicity of leachates from Florida municipal solid waste landfills using a battery-of-tests approach. Environ Toxicol 2002;17(3): 258–66.
[29] Agency for Toxic Substances and Disease Registry. Pilot exposure assessment of schools sited on or near hazardous waste sites in brownfields communities. 2002. p. 3–4. Available at: http://www.atsdr.cdc.gov/HEC/HSPH/v1n1-2part3.html. Accessed June 8, 2006.
[30] West S, Jackson H, Geller RJ, et al. Injury prevention. In: Frumkin H, Geller RJ, Rubin IL, et al, editors. Safe and healthy school environments. New York: Oxford University Press; 2006. p. 104–22.
[31] Audi J, Geller RJ. Chemical exposures in and out of classroom. In: Frumkin H, Geller RJ, Rubin IL, et al, editors. Safe and healthy school environments. New York: Oxford University Press; 2006. p. 189–206.
[32] US Environmental Protection Agency. El Dorado Hills, Naturally occurring asbestos. 2006. Available at: http://www.epa.gov/Region9/toxic/noa/eldorado/index.html. Accessed May 29, 2006.
[33] Azizian MF, Nelson PO, Thayumanavan P, et al. Environmental impact of highway construction and repair materials on surface and ground waters. Case study: crumb rubber asphalt concrete. Waste Manag 2003;23(8):719–28.
[34] Butler MA, Burr G, Dankovic D, et al. Hazard review: health effects of occupational exposure to asphalt. National Institute of Occupational Safety and Health. 2000. Available at: http://www.cdc.gov/niosh/pdfs/01-110.pdf. Accessed May 22, 2006.
[35] Farfel MR, Orlova AO, Lees PS, et al. A study of urban housing demolitions as sources of lead in ambient dust: demolition practices and exterior dust fall. Environ Health Perspect 2003;111(9):1228–34.
[36] Pickrell JA, Hill JO, Carpenter RL, et al. In vitro and in vivo response after exposure to man-made mineral and asbestos insulation fibers. Am Ind Hyg Assoc J 1983;44(8):557–61.
[37] Van Metre PC, Mahler BJ. The contribution of particles washed from rooftops to contaminant loading to urban streams. Chemosphere 2003;52(10):1727–41.
[38] US Environmental Protection Agency, Office of Groundwater and Drinking Water. Drinking water in schools & child care facilities. 3Ts for reducing lead in drinking water in schools. 2006. Available at: http://www.epa.gov/safewater/schools/guidance.html#3ts. Accessed May 22, 2006.
[39] Art and Creative Materials Institute. Safety: what you need to know. ACM Inc, 2004. Available at: http://www.acminet.org/Safety.htm. Accessed June 8, 2006.
[40] Maxwell LE. Crowding, class size and school size. In: Frumkin H, Geller RJ, Rubin IL, et al, editors. Safe and healthy school environments. New York: Oxford University Press; 2006. p. 13–9.
[41] Evans GW. Learning and the physical environment. In: Falk JH, Dierking LD, editors. Public institutions for personal learning: establishing a research agenda. Washington, DC: American Association of Museums; 1994. p. 119–26.
[42] Rodin J. Density, perceived choice, and responses to controllable and uncontrollable outcomes. J Exp Soc Psychol 1976;12:564–78.
[43] Erwine B. Lighting. In: Frumkin H, Geller RJ, Rubin IL, et al, editors. Safe and healthy school environments. New York: Oxford University Press; 2006. p. 20–33.
[44] Heschong Mahone Group (HMG). Daylighting in schools: an investigation into the relationship between daylighting and human performance. San Francisco (CA): Pacific Gas and Electric Company; 1999. HMG Project No. 9803.

[45] Benya J, Heschong L, McGowan T, et al. Advanced lighting guidelines. White Salmon (WA): New Buildings Institute; 2003. Available at: http://www.newbuildings.org/lighting.htm. Accessed June 8, 2006.

[46] Jaakkola JJK. Temperature and humidity. In: Frumkin H, Geller RJ, Rubin IL, et al, editors. Safe and healthy school environments. New York: Oxford University Press; 2006. p. 46–57.

[47] Mendell MJ, Heath GA. Do indoor pollutants and thermal conditions in schools influence student performance? A critical review of the literature. Indoor Air 2005;15:27–52.

[48] Institute of Medicine, Committee on Damp Indoor Spaces and Health. Damp indoor spaces and health. Washington, DC: National Academy of Sciences; 2004. p. 1–14.

[49] Maxwell LE. Noise. In: Frumkin H, Geller RJ, Rubin IL, et al, editors. Safe and healthy school environments. New York: Oxford University Press; 2006. p. 34–45.

[50] Sargent JW, Gidman MI, Humphreys MA, et al. The disturbance caused to school teachers by noise. Journal of Sound and Vibration 1980;70:557–72.

[51] Larson N, Story M. Nutrition at school: creating a healthy food environment. In: Frumkin H, Geller RJ, Rubin IL, et al, editors. Safe and healthy school environments. New York: Oxford University Press; 2006. p. 218–37.

[52] Perry CL, Bishop DB, Taylor GL, et al. A randomized school trial of environmental strategies to encourage fruit and vegetable consumption among children. Health Educ Behav 2004;31(1):65–76.

[53] Sneed J. Food safety. In: Frumkin H, Geller RJ, Rubin IL, et al, editors. Safe and healthy school environments. New York: Oxford University Press; 2006. p. 207–17.

[54] US Environmental Protection Agency. 2003. Pest control in the school environment: adopting integrated pest management. Available at: http://www.epa.gov/pesticides/ipm/brochure. Accessed June 8, 2006. Publication EPA-735-F-93-012.

[55] US Environmental Protection Agency. Integrated pest management for schools: a how-to manual. 2004. Available at: http://www.epa.gov/pesticides/ipm/schoolipm/index.html. Accessed June 8, 2006.

[56] Moore R. Playgrounds: a 150-year old model. In: Frumkin H, Geller RJ, Rubin IL, et al, editors. Safe and healthy school environments. New York: Oxford University Press; 2006. p. 86–103.

[57] Office of Technology Assessment. Risks to students in school. Washington, DC: US Government Printing Office; 1995. OTA-OTA-ENV-633.

[58] Tinsworth D, McDonald J. Special study: injuries and deaths associated with children's playground equipment. Bethesda (MD): U.S. Consumer Product Safety Commission; 2001.

[59] US Access Board. Americans with Disabilities Act (ADA) accessibility guidelines for play areas. 2000. Available at: http://www.access-board.gov/play/finalrule.htm. Accessed June 8, 2006.

[60] National Safe Kids Campaign. Facts about childhood sports injuries. Washington, DC: National Safe Kids Campaign; 2004. Available at:. http://www.usa.safekids.org/content_documents/Sports_facts.pdf. Accessed June 8, 2006.

[61] Consumer Product Safety Commission. CPSC Releases Study of protective equipment for baseball. Washington, DC; 1996. Available at: http://www.cpsc.gov/cpscpub/prerel/prhtml96/96140.html. Accessed May 23, 2006. Release #96-140.

[62] Marshall D. Safe and healthy sports environments. In: Frumkin H, Geller RJ, Rubin IL, et al, editors. Safe and healthy school environments. New York: Oxford University Press; 2006. p. 238–50.

[63] Delaney JS, Frankovich R. Head injuries and concussions in soccer. Clin J Sport Med 2005; 15:216–9.

[64] Almond CSD, Shin AY, Fortescue EB, et al. Hyponatremia among runners in the Boston Marathon. N Engl J Med 2005;352:1550–6.

[65] Maughan RJ, Leiper JB. Limitations to fluid replacement during exercise. Can J Appl Physiol 1999;24:173–87.

[66] Rehrer NJ. Fluid and electrolyte balance in ultra-endurance sport. Sports Med 2001;31: 701–15.

[67] Robertson HD, Tsai JC. Safe school travel. In: Frumkin H, Geller RJ, Rubin IL, et al, editors. Safe and healthy school environments. New York: Oxford University Press; 2006. p. 295–313.

[68] Speedy DB, Noakes TD, Schneider C. Exercise-associated hyponatremia: a review. Emerg Med 2001;13:17–27.

[69] Twerenbold R, Knechtie B, Kakebeeke TH, et al. Effects of different sodium concentrations in replacement fluids during prolonged exercise in women. Br J Sports Med 2003;37:300–3.

[70] Minehan MR, Riley MD, Burke LM. Effect of flavor and awareness of kilojoule content of drinks on preference and fluid balance in team sports. Int J Sport Nutr Exerc Metab 2002;12: 81–92.

[71] Dellinger AM, Beck LF. How risky is the commute to school? Deaths and injuries by transportation mode. TDR News 2005;237:22–5.

[72] Bellomo AJ. Emergency management. In: Frumkin H, Geller RJ, Rubin IL, et al, editors. Safe and healthy school environments. New York: Oxford University Press; 2006. p. 270–94.

ELSEVIER
SAUNDERS

Pediatr Clin N Am
54 (2007) 375–398

PEDIATRIC CLINICS
OF NORTH AMERICA

Environmental Health Disparities: Environmental and Social Impact of Industrial Pollution in a Community—the Model of Anniston, AL

I. Leslie Rubin, MD[a,b,c,d,*], Janice T. Nodvin, BA[a,b],
Robert J. Geller, MD[a,e,f], W. Gerald Teague, MD[a,e],
Brian L. Holtzclaw, BS[g], Eric I. Felner, MD[e,h]

[a]Emory Southeast Pediatric Environmental Health Specialty Unit, Atlanta, GA, USA
[b]Institute for the Study of Disadvantage and Disability, Atlanta, GA, USA
[c]Morehouse School of Medicine, Department of Pediatrics,
776 Windsor Parkway, Atlanta, GA 30342, USA
[d]The Team Centers and Developmental Pediatrics Specialists, Atlanta, GA, USA
[e]Emory University School of Medicine, Atlanta, GA, USA
[f]Georgia Poison Center, Atlanta, GA, USA
[g]United States Environmental Protection Agency, Region 4, Atlanta, GA, USA
[h]Pediatric Endocrinology, Hughes Spalding Children's Hospital, Atlanta, GA, USA

The health and well-being of children are critically dependent on the environment in which they live. This article explores the complex relationship between the environment in which a child lives and the environmental factors that can adversely affect health and development. It also examines how awareness of these adverse factors can be helpful in promoting optimal health for children through the societal infrastructures that deal with health, the environment, and social justice.

Paradigms in pediatric environmental health

Traditional pediatric care

Traditional pediatric practice focuses on an illness model in which the illness is caused by an agent. The pediatrician must diagnose the condition,

---

* Corresponding author. Department of Pediatrics, Morehouse School of Medicine, 776 Windsor Parkway, Atlanta, GA 30342.
   E-mail address: lrubi01@emory.edu (I.L. Rubin).

0031-3955/07/$ - see front matter © 2007 Elsevier Inc. All rights reserved.
doi:10.1016/j.pcl.2007.01.007

pediatric.theclinics.com

identify the causative agent, and treat the child by eradicating the cause and treating the symptoms to restore good health.

Pediatric environmental health

The term "pediatric environmental health" suggests that the pathologic agent is to be found in the environment and that the community, which includes pediatricians, public health practitioners and other responsible parties, must treat the child and must also seek to remove the offending agent from the environment to avoid further effects on the child in question or on other vulnerable children.

Disparities in environmental health

The term "environmental health disparities" suggests that there are groups of children who live in communities where there is a disproportionate exposure to certain environmental factors that can adversely affect the health and well-being of the children and that society at large has the responsibility to recognize the impact of these environmental factors and advocate on behalf of the children to promote more secure and healthier environments for the children and their families and thus effectively reduce health disparities.

Environmental justice

"Environmental justice" is both a concept and an approach to leverage existing laws to address environmental health disparities. The US Environmental Protection Agency (EPA) defines environmental justice as "the fair treatment and meaningful involvement of all people regardless of race, color, national origin, or income with respect to the development, implementation, and enforcement of environmental laws, regulations, and policies" (http://www.epa.gov/compliance/basics/ejbackground.html). This concept may be used to advocate on behalf of people who live in low-income and minority communities that are overburdened with adverse environmental factors and are underserved. Solutions to advance environmental justice have included conceptual, legal, and public policy mechanisms, as well as new strategies, models, and partnerships.

The pediatrician has a unique opportunity and responsibility to improve the quality of life of children who live in minority and low-income communities where they suffer disproportionate from adverse environmental impacts. The pediatrician can provide environmental education and support to families, school personnel, and other professional and lay individuals and organizations that come in contact with children. Advocacy is an active process in which pediatricians, having identified obstacles and barriers to the health and well-being of children, develop and promote mechanisms to assure that the barriers will be overcome and that the children will be assured

improved access to health care, appropriate education, and the necessary social support systems to grow into healthy and successful adults.

This article explores the more complex relationship between the environment in which a child lives and the environmental factors that can adversely
affect health and development. It also examines the how awareness of these
adverse factors can be helpful in promoting health for the children through
the societal infrastructure that deals with health, the environment, and
social justice.

Children's environmental health

The fetus, infant, and child are vulnerable to physical, chemical, and
biologic agents that cause illness as well as to other elements of the environment in which they live, including social, economic and political factors. It
may be helpful to conceptualize the impact of environmental factors in terms
of susceptibility and vulnerability to biologic factors (such as genetic predisposition and pre-existing conditions) as well as social conditions. At a simple
level the child can be seen in a nested diagram that encompasses the family
and the community in which the child lives (Fig. 1), but in reality more
complex factors operate, and it is helpful to consider community health
and vulnerability as well as individual health and vulnerability (Fig. 2).

Environmental health disparities

Environmental health disparities are reflected in epidemiologic findings
demonstrating that the morbidity and mortality of certain environmental
health conditions are disproportionately found in population groups that
live in circumstances of social and economic disadvantage. In the United
States, these populations include portions of the African American community, portions of minority immigrant communities (currently often Hispanic),
and portions of the Native American community [1]. These population groups
have several elements in common:

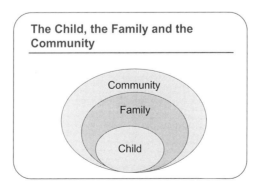

Fig. 1. The child, the family and the community.

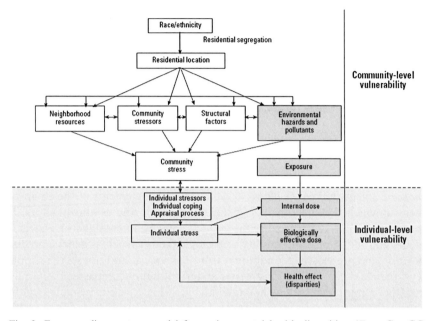

Fig. 2. Exposure-disease-stress model for environmental health disparities. (*From* Gee GC, Payne-Sturges DC. Environmental health disparities: a framework integrating psychosocial and environmental concepts. Environ Health Perspect 2004;112:1646. Published online 2004 August 16. doi: 10.1289/ehp.7074.)

1. Their financial resources are limited (resulting in limited choices as to where they can live).
2. They may have limited educational attainment and/or limited language skills for the marketplace and therefore have limited employment opportunities.
3. They may have limited social capital as far as empowerment and advocacy are concerned.
4. They are at the mercy of the low tax base of their place of residence, so that community and social resources are limited.
5. They may fear and distrust the established authority figures.

These factors may operate in a pattern that perpetuates the disparities. Fig. 3 presents a hypothetical formulation of the relationships between environmental factors and health. This figure is based on the Cycle of Disadvantage and Disability [2], which was constructed around a similar set of circumstances.

There are three major components to looking at health care disparities from an environmental perspective:

• Communities and neighborhoods: These factors look directly at the physical, chemical, and infrastructural elements within the immediate environment.

Cycle of Environmental Health Disparities

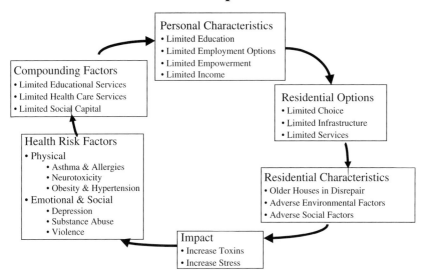

Fig. 3. Cycle of environmental health disparities (*Adapted from* Rubin IL, Crocker AC. Medical care for children and adults with developmental disabilities. 2nd edition. Baltimore (MD): Paul H Brookes; 2006. p. 231.)

- The social and cultural context: These factors look more broadly at the prevailing social structure, culture, and less tangible elements in an environment.
- Health care access for low income populations: Although this element may not be viewed readily as relevant to the environment, it is critically relevant to the environment in which the child lives; the access to appropriate preventive and therapeutic interventions has a profound influence on the health and well-being of children.

Communities and neighborhoods

In his review entitled "Dwelling Disparities," Hood [3] describes the adverse elements in neighborhoods and communities that have an impact on culture and lifestyle. Poorer communities are more likely to have liquor stores, fast-food places, and convenience stores but are less likely to have supermarkets and restaurants. The houses are more likely to be old and poorly maintained. Violence is more likely to be a part of the day-to-day life, creating fear among the residents and preventing the children from going outside to play and exercise safely, thus keeping them indoors and, most likely, watching television.

In many neighborhoods and communities, traffic patterns and construction projects create noise and air pollution that is disproportionately greater than can be found in more affluent neighborhoods. In addition, the poorer neighborhoods are less likely to have safe parks for children to play and open green spaces for recreation and relaxation [4,5].

Social and cultural context

Adverse economic factors affect individual and family health and well-being. They also can affect the social fabric of life and impact communities, community resources, and, most significantly, community cohesion. Psychosocial stress may be the vulnerability factor that links social conditions with environmental hazards. Gee and Payne-Sturges [6] posit that stress operates indirectly as well as directly in causing illness. They also suggest that residential segregation leads to differential experiences of community stress, exposure to pollutants, and access to community resources. When not counterbalanced by resources, stressors may lead to heightened vulnerability to environmental hazards. Recognition of these factors offers the opportunity to address the practical and emotional factors that cause diseases and disorders and also the stress that operates significantly in both the etiology and the treatment and management of the condition or conditions. The theoretic principle is to provide information, understanding, support, and empowerment, thereby reducing the stress and enhancing the personal and social circumstances for the individuals, families, and communities. These interventions can be implemented at a personal level as well as at a societal level through major public health and social campaigns [7,8].

Although poverty plays a significant role in determining the physical aspects of the environment, such as the location of the community and its infrastructure, there can be great diversity in the social and cultural characteristics of the community. The constellation of families, the organization of the community, and the prevailing values of the community play a large role in determining individual, family, and community well-being; and in some situations positive factors such as social cohesion may counteract the adverse environmental factors, particularly those of stress. The concept of social capital is helpful in understanding the impact of these factors on the health of individuals and population groups [9,10]. A study of poor and disadvantaged neighborhoods in Chicago between 1980 and 1986 found the rates of child abuse were two to three times higher in neighborhoods that were more socially disorganized and lacked social coherence than in more socially cohesive neighborhoods [9]. Low-income communities that are characterized as being unhelpful, unfair, and distrustful demonstrate a higher infant mortality [10]; in contrast, children from low-income areas that have high levels of social capital are less likely to drop out of school and are more likely to do well academically and socially [11,12].

Health care access for low-income populations

The socioeconomic and sociocultural aspects of the families who have low income and live in low-income communities are factors to consider in examining health care disparities in relation to environmental health disparities. Limited access to affordable and convenient health care significantly affects the health and well-being of children in poorer communities. Access to quality health care is not merely an issue of the availability of health care centers, but also the quality of the health care encounter. A report by the Commonwealth Fund on disparities in primary care by income revealed that adults in the United States who had below-average incomes had more negative experiences in obtaining access to primary care, were more likely to go without care because of costs, and were more likely to have negative experiences in the doctor–patient relationship [13]. This experience of adults relates directly to the health care children receive, because it is the adult parents who decide, on the basis of their experience, how to use the health care delivery system for their children. A study of African American and Latino households in urban public housing communities in the Los Angeles area revealed that these children were two to four times more likely to suffer from chronic physical and mental conditions than the general population. The common chronic conditions reported by parents for one or more children in their households were asthma, eye/vision problems, dental problems, attention-deficit hyperactivity disorder (ADHD), and depression [14]. A combination of factors currently inherent in the health care delivery system is weighted against individuals and families who have limited or no insurance, who have limited access to transportation, and who may not have a primary care pediatrician or medical home [15].

The pediatrician and environmental health disparities

The pediatrician's traditional role is the promotion of child health by preventing disease, by conducting regular and appropriate health and developmental screening to identify and treat conditions early, and by treating acute and chronic illnesses that arise. In providing health care for children who live in adverse environmental circumstances, the pediatrician is challenged by factors that increase the risk of adverse effects on health, growth, and development and by factors that prevent children from having access to adequate and consistent health care screening, prevention, and treatment of acute conditions and management of chronic conditions. The traditional notion that a causative agent results in illness that has corresponding curative treatment addresses only part of the pediatrician's responsibility in caring for children who have chronic conditions or who live in environments that place them at increased risk for adverse health effects. In order to improve the health and well-being of all children, pediatricians must explore the environmental factors that affect the health of their young patients, suggest ways in which they can be mitigated, and advocate improvements in environmental conditions on behalf of the children and their communities.

Clinical conditions and environmental factors

Some environmental health conditions have a clear and direct effect on health. In other conditions the mechanisms may be more complex. The next section reviews and discusses four clinical conditions of childhood, each of which examines the relationship between the environment and the specific health condition from a different perspective.

Lead toxicity

In the past, lead toxicity was a problem that affected all populations of children. Although the elimination of lead from gasoline, paint, and ceramics has dramatically reduced the prevalence of lead toxicity, it has become increasingly clear that children from different social, economic, ethnic, and geographic backgrounds have different risks of exposure and hence have different likelihoods of having an elevated blood lead level. The most vulnerable populations in the United States today are low-income African American and Hispanic American children who live in older urban housing. In the 1991–1994 National Health and Nutrition Examination Survey (NHANES III) data, risk of having a blood lead level between 10 and 20 μg/dL was 2.4 times greater (95% confidence interval [CI], 1.2–4.8) for children receiving Medicaid than for children not receiving Medicaid, and those living in poverty had 2.7 times the risk of more affluent children (95% CI, 1.2–6.0). Non-Hispanic black children were 7.3 times more likely to have a blood lead level between 10 and 20 μg/dL than non-Hispanic white children (95% CI, 2.4–15.4) [16].

In some communities, legal mandates have been created to force reduction in lead found in housing. In other communities, such legislation does not exist, and the only option available to the family may be to move to a different residence. Federal law does require that every residential renter and every home buyer be informed of the lead status of the property before signing the contract to rent or purchase, and failure to do so carries substantial penalties. This statute often can be used as leverage to encourage clean up of lead-contaminated housing units, as is the current strategy in the State of Georgia.

Air pollution and asthma

Asthma is the most common chronic disease of children, is most prevalent in the very young, and affects between 5% and 7% of preadolescent children in the United States [17]. Nationally, asthma is significantly more prevalent in African Americans and Hispanic Americans than the general population. Poverty and minority ethnic status disproportionately increase asthma morbidity and mortality in the pediatric population, especially children from the inner city [18].

A 1996 report from the federal Centers for Disease Control and Prevention shows hospitalization and deaths rates from asthma increasing for persons 25 years or less. The greatest increases occurred among African Americans, who are two to six times more likely than whites to die from asthma and three to four times more likely to be hospitalized for asthma. Explanations for these disparities do point to clear environmental factors, but it is equally evident that the association is more complex and multifactorial. In New York, people living within a specified distance of noxious land uses were 66% more likely to be hospitalized for asthma, 30% more likely to be poor, and 13% more likely to be a member of a minority than those outside the zones [19]. Pediatric emergency department visits at Atlanta's Grady Memorial Hospital increased by one third when the ground level ozone levels exceeded federal monitoring standards. The asthma rate among African American children in this study is 26% higher than the asthma rate among whites. In a randomized telephone survey conducted in Georgia in 2000, the prevalence of asthma was negatively associated with the level of self-reported household income (Fig. 4) [20]. This disparity may be related to housing practices, exposure to airborne pollutants resulting from residence in the inner city, access to prescription medication, the quality of medical care, and/or other factors not identified. Among Georgia children whose medical care was financed by Medicaid [21], the prevalence of physician-diagnosed asthma based on claims data

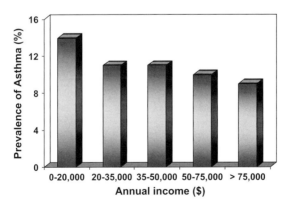

Fig. 4. Prevalence of asthma versus self-reported household income from a randomized survey of Georgia families. (*Adapted From* Mellinger-Birdsong AK, Powell KE, Iatridis T. 2000 Georgia Asthma Report. Georgia Department of Human Resources, Division of Public Health, Chronic Disease, Injury, and Environmental Epidemiology Section. December, 2000. Publication number DPH00.65H.)

was equally high in health districts with low population densities as in urban districts.

Obesity

Obesity in children, adolescents, and adults has reached epidemic proportions, with minorities being affected disproportionately [22]. The prevalence of adolescent obesity has increased significantly in only 5 years: from 10.5% (in 1988 to 1994) to 15.5% (in 1999 to 2000). Obesity was significantly more prevalent among African American adolescents (23.6%) than in white adolescents (12.7%) [22–25]. According to the NHANES III survey, approximately 22% of African American children 6 to 17 years of age are obese [26]. Obesity has approximately the same association with chronic illness as does 20 years of aging, and obesity has an even stronger association with reduction in health-related quality of life and the health care costs of smoking, problem drinking, and poverty [27,28].

Complications of obesity include increased incidence of type 2 diabetes, hypertension, cardiovascular disease, sleep apnea, asthma, and gallbladder disease in children [29–38]. During the past 20 years, the proportion of hospital discharges for obesity and obesity-related problems in children 6 to 17 years of age increased dramatically [39].

Obesity and diabetes are becoming more common clinical and public health problems in all segments of society; but they occur with increased frequency among African American and Hispanic immigrant populations. The environments in which these children live and the social and economic stresses they face play a significant role in the etiology and epidemiology of these conditions. The neighborhoods, schools, and the homes where these children reside play a vital role in their development of obesity.

The ability for children to engage in physical activity depends on the physical design and quality of their neighborhood [40]. For safety reasons, parents may restrict their children's participation in outdoor activities by using television and easy access to snacks. The lack of well-developed parks and recreational facilities in low-income urban environments also limits children's opportunities for physical activity. In low-income communities, family work schedules and lack of money and car availability make it difficult for parents to transport children to recreational activities [41].

Schools offer opportunities for improving children's nutrition and increasing their physical activity. Unfortunately, many inner-city schools are unable to take advantage of these opportunities [42]. Many schools offer a wide variety of foods that do not meet nutritional standards but generate substantial revenue for the schools [43]. Many of these inner-city schools, attempting to improve scholastic performance, replace physical activity with classes focused on academic improvement.

The home environment also is a major factor contributing to the increased obesity in low-socioeconomic populations. Knowledge of nutritional requirements and health may be limited, with television advertisements providing most of the ideas about eating habits. The ability to provide a healthy, balanced diet also is compromised by the family's economic status: poorer neighborhoods are more likely to have convenience stores instead of supermarkets, and the food choices are limited, more expensive, and less likely to be fresh [3,44–47].

Any strategy addressing childhood obesity must include interventions targeted at the child's environment and its psychosocial stressors.

Attention-deficit hyperactivity disorder and learning disabilities

Although ADHD has reached epidemic proportions in the United States, there are health care and environmental health disparities in the diagnosis and management of this condition that have a serious effect on a child's potential for future employment and hence financial security and success. ADHD is more likely to be identified and treated in children from more affluent and resourceful families and neighborhoods [48]. In Los Angeles, more than 1500 elementary school students were screened for ADHD [49], and the predictors of help-seeking steps among the high-risk group (23.6% of the total) and parent-identified barriers to care among children with unmet needs for ADHD care (5.5% of the total) were evaluated. Although 88% of the identified group was recognized as having a problem, only 39% were evaluated, only 32% received the diagnosis of ADHD, and only 23% received treatment. The families of white children were twice as likely to take active help-seeking steps as the families of African American children. For the children who had unmet needs for ADHD care, poverty predicted lower treatment rates and was associated with the most pervasive barriers.

These disparities in seeking help for ADHD are related both to family and cultural factors and to external factors such as teacher and school attitudes and the accessibility and availability of appropriate pediatric care [48]. A survey exploring cultural differences between African American and white respondents found that African American families were more likely than whites to be unfamiliar with ADHD, its treatment, or its complications and often had concerns about misdiagnosis. In addition, the survey found that African Americans believed that they were diagnosed as having ADHD more often than whites because of stereotyping and biases in assessment and diagnosis and were less likely to be treated [49].

Another area of concern related to ADHD is the higher prevalence of lead toxicity among children living in poorer environments. As the understanding of lead toxicity has progressed, the acceptable blood lead level for children has dropped dramatically, the appreciation of the effects of lead toxicity in children has become refined, and attention is being paid to the more subtle but still significant manifestations such as learning disabilities and behavior problems [50–52]. Children with excessive exposure to lead also may attend older, poorly maintained inner-city schools that have both environmental and psychosocial factors that adversely affect a child's ability to focus and learn.

In children from neighborhoods where academic achievement and success at school are not part of the prevailing pressures, ADHD and learning disabilities may go undiagnosed or untreated, resulting in school failure with grade retention, graduation with an unsatisfactory and limited education, or dropping out of school (Table 1) [53]. An increased dropout rate is associated with a reduced likelihood of employment and an increased likelihood of substance abuse, sexual promiscuity, teenage pregnancy, and teen-age male violence (with the associated morbidity as well as increased involvement with the law and possible incarceration). The outcomes of the teenage pregnancies are more likely to be associated with prematurity or low birth weight infants [54]. If the teen-aged mother uses cigarettes, alcohol, or other illegal substances, the fetus is more likely to have neurodevelopmental consequences of intrauterine exposure or consequences of prematurity (Table 2). Once the infant is born, the young mother is less likely to be able to care for the child; emotional and social factors may result in neglect or abuse of the child and rearing of the child in a single-parent or nonparental home. This cycle of circumstances serves to perpetuate and even aggravate the adverse economic, social, and emotional environment and result in greater degrees of morbidity and an increase in mortality [2].

Case study: Anniston, Alabama

Anniston is a town of approximately 25,000 residents in northeast Alabama. In 2000, the racial composition was approximately 54% white, 44% black, and 2% other. Anniston was founded in the late nineteenth century as a mining and iron-producing town. Similar foundry-, military-, and chemical-based industries continued to locate in the city. In the late

Table 1
Cognitive and educational effects of poverty on children

Indicator	Children who are poor (%)	Children who are not poor (%)	Ratio poor/ not poor
Developmental delay	5.0	3.8	1.3
Learning disability	8.3	6.1	1.4
Grade retention	28.8	14.1	2.0
Ever expelled or suspended	12.1	6.1	2.0
High school dropout rate in 1994	21.0	9.6	2.2
Not employed or in school at age 24 years	15.9	8.	1.9

Data from Wood D. Effect of Child and Family Poverty on Child Health in the United States. Pediatrics 2003;112:707–11.

Table 2
Risk of adverse child outcomes and environmental conditions associated with poverty status

Child outcomes	Risk for poor children relative to not-poor children
Lead poisoning	3.5
Birth to unmarried teenager	3.1
Short-stay hospital episode	2.0
Grade repetition and high school dropout	2.0
Low birth weight	1.7
Mortality	1.7
Learning disability	1.4
Parent report of emotional or behavior problem that lasted 3 months or more	1.3
Socioeconomic status mediators	
Child abuse and neglect	6.8
Depression	2.3
Victim of violent crimes	2.2
Substance abuse	1.9

Adapted from Neurons to Neighborhoods: The Science of Early Childhood Development. Institute of Medicine; 2000. p. 274.

1920s, one chemical plant began biphenyl production. From the 1930s through the 1970s, more than 1.5 billion pounds of polychlorinated biphenyls (PCBs) were manufactured in the United States by only two plants, one of which was in Anniston. During its 42-year operational history, the Anniston PCB plant disposed of hazardous waste at adjacent properties: its West End landfill (until 1961) and the South landfill (until 1988). In addition, some product was given to local people for termite control and fencepost treatment. In the 1970s and 1980s, PCB was detected in downstream fish, floodplains, and sediment; by the early 1990s the state Public Health Department issued the first fish consumption advisory warning people to avoid eating all fish caught in local downstream waterways [55].

In February 2000, the Centers for Disease Control Agency for Toxic Substance and Disease Registry (ATSDR) released a *Health Consultation on the Evaluation of Soil, Blood and Air Data from Anniston, Alabama* that summarized data available at that time [56,57]. The analysis showed widespread PCB-affected soil in Anniston and deemed exposure to such soil a public health hazard. The PCB-contaminated air was deemed an indeterminate public hazard because the unknown effects of long-term exposure and unknown home concentrations; although PCB air samples of the top five monitors were 20 times higher than the background air samples (Table 3).

Blood testing confirmed a pattern of human PCB exposure that identified Anniston as one of the most heavily exposed communities in the nation. These levels were much higher than the mean serum PCB levels of 0.9 to

Table 3
Number of persons sampled with blood PCB levels above 10, 20, and 100 μg/L or parts per billion, Anniston, Alabama

Of all persons (N = 2966)	Number	Percentage of total
Number of persons above 10 μg/L	1037	34.9
Number of persons above 20 μg/L	521	17.5
Number of persons above 100 μg/L	41	1.4

Data from Agency for Toxic Substances and Disease Registry. Toxicological profile for PCBs. Atlanta (GA): Agency for Toxic Substances and Disease Registry; 2000. p. 557–60; Canady R. Health consultation; evaluation of soil, blood, and air data from Anniston, Alabama. Atlanta (GA): Agency for Toxic Substances and Disease Registry; 2000.

1.5 ppb found in recent years in unexposed populations [56]. The ATSDR [56,57] stated

> Most of the high PCB levels [ie, those over 100 μg/L] were in persons over 50 years of age at the time their blood was sampled. However, 346 persons under the age of 50 had greater than 10 μg/L PCB, including one 38-year-old person with a blood PCB level of 124 μg/L. Two children less than 6 years of age had blood PCB levels between 10 and 20 μg/L, and one 12-year-old had a blood PCB level of 26 μg/L.

Community reaction

When the citizens of Anniston realized their vulnerability to the adverse health effects of the PCBs, they perceived a situation of environmental injustice and started on the path of litigation. Their concerns were supported by publications such as the *U.S. News and World Report* article, "Kids at Risk" [58], which highlighted Anniston as having a challenging mixture of environmental exposures. Even the EPA identified the PCB problems as serious enough to warrant the creation of an Anniston PCB Superfund Site, a designated area with a high risk to human health and the environment. The citizens were somewhat relieved that this designation qualified their community for widespread sampling investigations over large tracts of residential and commercial properties and for short- and long-term cleanups [1].

In late 2000 the EPA Region 4 office provided funds and collaborated with the Southeast Pediatric Environmental Health Specialty Unit (PEHSU) to provide information and technical support to residents of Anniston and to raise local pediatricians' awareness of and understanding about the potential adverse effects of environmental toxins. The original scope of that request focused on continuing medical education sessions for Anniston physicians. Through this process, representatives of the Southeast PEHSU met concerned physicians and learned about programs for children and other community resources. They began to expand their contacts and met with community action groups, local elected officials, agencies dealing with children, representatives from schools, and other community members active in working with children, especially children at risk, to become better acquainted with the situation and to determine if there were other ways the PEHSU could be of assistance.

Several observations emerged from these meetings: a) the disparities in exposure to pollution, b) concern about the health of children, and c) the need to mobilize resources for children in Anniston.

Disparities in exposure to pollution

It became abundantly clear at an early stage of the consultation that the patterns of PCB exposure in Anniston affected African American residents disproportionately more than white residents. The former PCB chemical facility and its waste sites were located in West Anniston, the predominantly African American and poorer part of the city (Fig. 5). This location had the

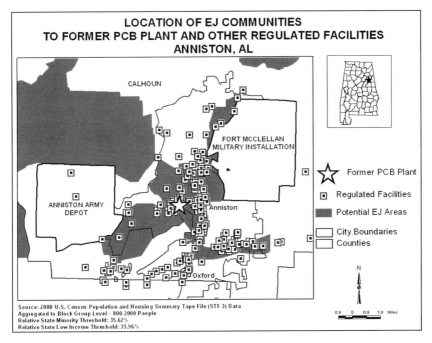

Fig. 5. Map of greater Anniston demonstrating the close proximity of Environmental Justice (EJ) communities with respect to the former polychlorinated biphenyls (PCB) plant and other environmentally regulated manufacturing facilities The EJ areas are defined using Environmental Protection Agency (EPA) Region 4 thresholds for significant low-income (35.96%) and/or minority populations (35.62%) in Alabama. GIS map: location of EJ communities to former PCB plant and other regulated facilities using data at time of EPA Superfund intervention in 2000, namely: 2000 US Census data; 2000 Housing Summary Tape File (STF3) data; EPA Region 4 environmental justice demographic thresholds for minority and low-income populations for Alabama; and 2000 Environmental Regulated Facility data, August 2006. (*From* Holtzclaw B, Carbonaro S, Rigger D, et al. Environmental justice at the Anniston PCB/lead superfund sites (AL). Presented at the US EPA Office of Site Remediation and Enforcement. Washington, DC, June 3, 2003.)

distinct effect of polarizing the community along racial and economic lines. The leader of the largest of the community activist groups, David Baker, a member of Community Against Pollution (CAP), was particularly outspoken and determined and was responsible for hiring a nationally renowned African American litigator, Johnnie Cochran, Jr. CAP, a grassroots, non-profit organization, was formed to give a voice to people living at risk from PCBs. It was not difficult to understand the atmosphere of tension and mistrust that emerged. The animosity and tensions operated in both directions, resulting in racial polarization to the point of impasse.

While the factories were operating at full steam in West Anniston, there was employment, a good tax base, and a sense of economic well-being. Once the manufacturing plants began to close, and the pollution had been identified, there was a sense of abandonment coupled with a negative impact on employment and family income and a sense of injustice from the legacy of pollution. Despite the profound emotional and social implications resulting in a mixture of anger and diminishing hope, the idea of obtaining justice though litigation and the expectation of a financial settlement that would right the wrongs kept the momentum positive and the hope alive.

Concern about the health of children

There was widespread concern among family members and community representatives that the impact of the toxins increased the likelihood of birth defects, increased learning and behavior problems among school-age children, and increased substance abuse and behavior problems that resulted in an increase in teen pregnancies.

One of the greatest challenges was to respond to the community's concern about the health, growth, and development of its children and its perception that the PCBs had caused the problems the children were experiencing. Although the children had evident problems, it was not possible to link the specific concerns about the children clearly to PCB exposure. Problems in attributing causality included the facts that not all the children had been tested and that the community was in litigation and the lawyers had cautioned the citizens about becoming involved in efforts at resolution.

Although specific information about the health and developmental status of the children of Anniston was limited, Alabama trailed most states on several birth measures. Alabama ranked among the bottom 10 states in four of the eight measures of a healthy start to life: teen-aged births, repeat teen-aged births, low birth weight births, and preterm births. Moreover, the key indicators of infant health for 1999 ranked Alabama among the bottom 10% in the percentage of total births to teens, percentage of total births to mothers with less than 12 years of education, and percentage of births that were low birth weight (less than 5.5 lbs) infants [59].

While these data bode poorly for developmental benchmarks for children in Alabama in general, the situation in Anniston was likely to be even worse, because of the documented toxins in the environment and the poor social and economic climate in the community. A Health Care Needs Assessment done in Calhoun County (the location of Anniston) in 2001 by the Public Affairs Research Council of Alabama revealed that the people of the county reported fair or poor general health status 34% of the time (compared with 19% reported for Alabama overall and a United States average of 12%). In addition, residents of Calhoun County reported mental health concerns more often than Alabamans overall, who in turn had such concerns more often than the general United States population [60].

The next step was to work with the community to address its concerns and to help develop mechanisms to improve the situation for the children and their families.

Mobilization of resources for children in Anniston

The town of Anniston had an array of local and regional community resources, including colleges, school system officials, dedicated elected officials, a thriving business community, a community foundation, and a sizeable medical community. These stakeholders, however, had not yet come together in any common forum. Although community agencies often operate independently despite their common purposes, the situation in Anniston had the added complication of racial polarization, fractiousness, and ongoing litigation.

A steering committee was established, chaired by the mayor of Anniston and consisting of representatives from a cross section of the Anniston community—business people, faculty from local colleges, representatives from the community activist group, educators, and local physicians. Over the next 2 years the steering committee was able to build trust among all the parties and to help articulate a shared vision of how to respond to the challenges of child development in Anniston. In mid-2001 the steering committee established a clear agenda and a clear timeline. Both were reflected in the name that the project adopted—*Vision 2020, for the Children of Anniston*—because, "By the year 2020, there will be a record number of young men and women graduating from high school who go on to colleges across the country." Vision 2020 and its board of directors became emblematic of the resilience of the community, its ability to mobilize its resources, the willingness of the diverse aspects of the community to work together, and the community's dedication to making sure that the children of Anniston receive an education they deserve to prepare for the future. In March 2003, in recognition of the success of Vision 2020 and the other efforts, the Federal Interagency Working Group on Environmental Justice designated Anniston as one of 15 EPA Revitalization Demonstration Projects [55].

Although in Anniston the toxic exposures of concern were chemicals from a manufacturing plant that posed health hazards to children and adults alike, the real issues were much more complex. The reality that the affected population was the poorer citizens, who also were largely African American, brought a different dimension to the fore: the realization that being poor increased the likelihood of exposure to environmental toxins and that, once toxic exposure has occurred and been identified, the process of treatment and rehabilitation is more challenging because of the complexity of the social and economic factors (see Fig. 3).

Environmental justice

To understand better the inequities encountered in Anniston, it is necessary to examine the conceptual and practical aspects of the term "environmental justice." There is a growing body of multidisciplinary research documenting disproportionate impacts of pollution and toxins on people who live in circumstances of social and economic disadvantage.

Gee and Payne-Sturges" [6] stress-exposure-disease model (see Fig. 2) provides the conceptual framework to explain environmental justice. They propose that the leading reason certain communities with specific social, economic, cultural, ethnic, or minority characteristics face stresses, such as living with a myriad of polluting facilities, is highly correlated with the location of residential housing and comes with differential exposure to health risks [6,61].

The roots of modern environmental justice emerged more than 25 years ago from fragmented communities that were seeking resolution of their local environmental disputes and organized a collective movement to confront challenges to fair and equal protection from environmental and health hazards. These early years of the environmental justice movement focused on hazardous waste sites and other polluting facilities that were located in or near poor and minority neighborhoods. In 1979, the African American community of North Hollywood in Houston, Texas, filed suit to prevent the establishment of a solid-waste landfill. In 1982 the predominantly African American community of Warren County in North Carolina protested the establishment of a PCB landfill [62,63]. These incidents brought together the environmental and civil rights movements, a coalition that resulted in the landmark study, "Toxic Wastes and Race in the United States" [64]. This report introduced the term "environmental racism" into the lexicon to make the point that the groups of people suffering from the environmental hazards were of minority status, specifically African American. Since those early beginnings, a series of social, political, and legal actions and achievements have helped the concept of Environmental Justice to develop. As consciousness of environmental conditions in low-income, people of color, and tribal communities grew, a more comprehensive set of issues came to the forefront that included toxicants, lead poisoning in housing, land use, brownfield sites, air quality, workplace health and safety, transportation, and economic development as well as issues of race and poverty [65].

The 1992 Presidential Executive Order 12898, "Federal Actions to Address Environmental Justice in Minority Populations and Low-Income Populations" was a testament to growing national public concern and emerging scientific research on these environmental inequities [66]. This order attempted to address environmental injustice by leveraging existing federal laws and regulations. In addition, although the United States Constitution created a representative government, society has not yet provided equal access to decision-making processes, particularly for low-income and minority communities, that would ensure a healthy environment in which to live, learn, play, and work.

Thus, environmental justice incorporates two major societal components [63,65]:

1. Knowledge of the impact of adverse environmental factors on the health and well-being of individuals and communities
2. An extension of the civil rights movement, which addresses the situation in which groups of individuals encounter discrimination for whatever reason—be it socioeconomic, ethnic, racial, religious, or political

In the case of Anniston, the nonprofit citizen group, CAP, became the voice by which people living in the PCB-contaminated community could participate in those decisions. This voice played a critical role in the EPA's decision to take a stronger position by designating a Superfund Site, and that same voice was instrumental in forming the Children's Health Initiative in Anniston [1].

More and more communities facing issues of environmental justice are shifting from a focus on problem identification to a focus on problem resolution. Despite great obstacles such as limited human, technical, financial, social, and political capital, these affected communities are determined to affect positive change on behalf of healthy communities.

Charles Lee [63], a 25-year veteran in the environmental justice movement who also leads the EPA's National Environmental Justice Advisory Council, presents a way to examine the core concepts that embody environmental justice. For the clinician, it provides a familiar framework that mirrors the paradigm of the clinical approach to a problem: a knowledge base for the treatment that leads to a suggested treatment approach:

1. The meaning of disproportionate impacts, a concept originally centered on disproportionate exposure and since expanded to encompass cumulative environmental hazards, vulnerability, inequities in regulatory enforcement, and disparities in socioeconomic status, power, and health
   a. This element describes the situation in which the health and well-being of people living in specific communities are at risk or adversely affected by environmental factors that exist at an unusual, unreasonable, and unacceptable level, and the community has relatively limited resources to deal with them.

   b. In the Anniston case presentation, the contributing factors were the presence of chemical pollutants in the residential areas of predominantly African American and poor people who lived near manufacturing plants (see Fig. 5).
2. The legal, public policy, and research challenges inherent in the concept of environmental justice, particularly those related to integrating civil rights and social justice concepts into an environmental law paradigm
   a. This element refers to the emergence of conceptual, legal, and public policy mechanisms over the past 2 to 3 decades to provide communities with opportunities to change a situation by removing the environmental hazards and improving the health and well-being of its citizens.
   b. In the Anniston case, the EPA, the Agency for Toxic Substances and Disease Registry (ATSDR), and the legal system presented these challenges. The members of the community who became active and vocal and who took the initiative were able to change the status quo.
3. The community-based collaborative problem-solving strategies and tools needed to address the interrelated environmental, health, economic, and social concerns of disadvantaged, underserved, and overburdened communities
   a. This element is the one that begins to look at the question. "Where do we go from here?" Because of the underlying complexities of the situation, the resolution clearly requires a broad-based and collaborative approach. The environmentally and economically distressed community coordinates the existing local, tribal, state, and/or federal initiatives and resources (human, technical, legal, institutional, and financial) to help with revitalization. A comprehensive solution to address economic and social factors such as housing, transportation, economic development, job creation, green space, and recreation will take dynamic and proactive partnerships [67].
   b. In the Anniston case, through the Children's Health Initiative of Vision 2020, it was possible to assemble representatives from a variety of community services and agencies, with outside consultants used as appropriate to address the needs of the children and to begin to develop programs to meet their needs [68].

As the environmental justice paradigm has matured, it has become more holistic and integrative, increasingly viewing individual and community health as a product of physical, social, cultural, and spiritual elements. This approach aligns with the World Health Organization's view of community health as a positive concept that "encompasses all the environmental, social and economic resources as well as the emotional and physical capacities that enable people in a geographic area to realize their aspirations and satisfy their needs" [69].

Summary

Children's environmental health reflects the sum of environmental factors that affect the health of children at many levels, from exposures to specific toxic substances, to the physical and infrastructural elements in families and communities, and to social, economic, and cultural aspects of society. The children who are most vulnerable to environmental hazards are those who live in circumstances of social and economic disadvantage. In the context of their environment, the differential vulnerability of children to health-related factors in specified population groups can be viewed under the lens of environmental health disparities. The social and political systems that are in place to address and redress these environmental health disparities and the emerging legal precedents can be subsumed under the term "environmental justice."

Pediatricians who serve children from a variety of backgrounds, particularly those associated with poverty, minority status, and immigrant populations or from families who are otherwise unempowered or disenfranchised, need to be aware of the environmental factors and their impact on the health of the children. Each child needs to be seen in the broader community context, and exploration of the possible causes of childhood diseases and disorders needs to be particularly deliberate and searching. Likewise, the approach to treatment, rehabilitation, and management must take into consideration the family constellation, parent education and employment, other family members involved, financial and insurance coverage, the condition of the house, home, and neighborhood, and other social and economic factors.

In this context, the American Academy of Pediatrics [15] promotes the Medical Home concept, which underscores the need to provide comprehensive and coordinated health care for children that is community based and culturally sensitive [15]. In providing such care, the pediatrician can help mitigate disparities in environmentally induced illnesses by correcting health injustices and by helping prevent these adverse health conditions from arising.

References

[1] Holtzclaw B, Carbonaro S, Rigger D, et al. Environmental justice at the Anniston PCB/lead superfund sites (AL). Presented at the US EPA Office of Site Remediation and Enforcement. Washington, DC, June 3, 2003.

[2] Rubin IL, Crocker AC. Medical care for children and adults with developmental disabilities. 2nd Edition. Baltimore (MD): Paul H Brookes; 2006.

[3] Hood Ernie. Focus: dwelling disparities. Environ Health Perspect 2005;113(5):A310–7.

[4] Apelberg BJ, Buckley TJ, White RH. Socioeconomic and racial disparities in cancer risk from air toxics in Maryland. Environ Health Perspect 2005;113(6):693–9.

[5] Brugge D, Leong A, Averbach AR, et al. An environmental health survey of residents in Boston Chinatown. J Immigr Health 2000;2:97–111.

[6] Gee GC, Payne-Sturges DC. Environmental health disparities: a framework integrating psychosocial and environmental concepts. Environ Health Perspect 2004;112:1645–53.

[7] Waterston T, Alperstein G, Stewart Brown S. Social capital: a key factor in child health inequalities. Arch Dis Child 2004;89:456–9.

[8] Weber R, Orsini D, Sullivan A, et al. Short-term temporal variation in PM 2.5 mass and chemical composition during the Atlanta supersite experiment, 1999. J Air Waste Manag Assoc 2003;53(1):84–91.

[9] Garbarino J, Kostelny K. Child maltreatment as a community problem. Child Abuse Negl 1992;16(4):455–64.

[10] Kawachi I, Kennedy BP, Lochner K, et al. Social capital, income inequality, and mortality. Am J Public Health 1997;87(9):1504–6.

[11] Runyan DK, Hunter WM, Socolar RR, et al. Children who prosper in unfavorable environments: the relationship to social capital. Pediatrics 1998;101(1 Pt 1):12–8.

[12] Sexton K. Sociodemographic aspects of human susceptibility to toxic chemicals: do class and race matter for realistic rick assessment?". Environ Toxicol Pharmacol 1997;4:267–9.

[13] Huynh PT, Schoen C, Osborn R, et al. The U.S. health care divide: disparities in primary care experiences by income. The Commonwealth Fund, 2006.

[14] Bazargan M, Calderon JL, Heslin KC, et al. A profile of chronic mental and physical conditions among African-American and Latino children in urban public housing. Ethn Dis 2005;15(4 Suppl 5): S5-S3-9.

[15] Tonniges TF, Palfrey JS. The Medical Home. Pediatrics 2004;113:1471–548.

[16] Bernard SM, McGeehin MA. Prevalence of blood lead levels ≥ 5 μg/dL among US children 1 to 5 years of age and socioeconomic and demographic factors associated with blood of lead levels 5 to 10 μg/dL, Third National Health and Nutrition Examination Survey, 1988–1994. Pediatrics 2003;112:1308–13.

[17] DeMeo DL, Weiss ST. Epidemiology. In: Barnes PJ, Drazen JM, Rennard S, et al, editors. Asthma and COPD. Amsterdam: Academic Press; 2002. p. 7–17.

[18] Persky VW, Slezak J, Contreras A, et al. Relationships of race and socioeconomic status with prevalence, severity, and symptoms of asthma in Chicago school children. Ann Allergy Asthma Immunol 1998;81:266–71.

[19] Maantay J. Asthma and air pollution in the Bronx: methodological and data considerations in using GIS for environmental justice and health research. Health & Place 2007; 13(1):32–56.

[20] Mellinger-Birdsong AK, Powell KE, Iatridis T. 2000 Georgia asthma report. Georgia Department of Human Resources, Division of Public Health publication #DPH00.65H. Georgia Department of Human Resources; 2000.

[21] Teague WG, Chapman K. A population-based study of disease prevalence, hospital admission rates, and physician prescribing behaviors in pediatric Medicaid enrollees with asthma. Am J Respir Crit Care Med 1999;159:A144.

[22] Dwyer JT, Stone EJ, Yang M, et al. Prevalence of marked overweight and obesity in a multiethnic pediatric population: findings from the Child and Adolescent Trial for Cardiovascular Health (CATCH) study. J Am Diet Assoc 2000;100:1149–56.

[23] Nieto FJ, Szklo M, Comstock GW. Childhood weight and growth rate as predictors of adult mortality. Am J Epidemiol 1992;136:201–13.

[24] Ogden CL, Flegal KM, Carroll MD, et al. Prevalence and trends in overweight among US children and adolescents, 1999–2000. JAMA 2002;288(14):1728–32.

[25] Peel JL, Tolbert PE, Klein M, et al. Ambient air pollution and respiratory emergency department visits. Epidemiology 2005;16:164–74.

[26] Troiano RP, Flegal KM, Kuczmarski RJ, et al. Overweight prevalence and trends for children and adolescents. The National Health and Nutrition Examination Surveys, 1963 to 1991. Arch Pediatr Adolesc Med 1995;149:1085–91.

[27] Sturm R. The effects of obesity, smoking, and drinking on medical problems and costs. Obesity outranks both smoking and drinking in its deleterious effects on health and health costs. Health Aff (Millwood) 2002;21:245–53.

[28] Sturm R, Wells KB. Does obesity contribute as much to morbidity as poverty or smoking? Public Health 2001;115:229–35.

[29] Must A, Spadano J, Coakley EH, et al. The disease burden associated with overweight and obesity. JAMA 1999;282:1523–9.

[30] Must A, Strauss RS. Risks and consequences of childhood and adolescent obesity. Int J Obes Relat Metab Disord 1999;23(Suppl 2):S2–11.

[31] Must A, Jacques PF, Dallal GE, et al. Long-term morbidity and mortality of overweight adolescents. A follow-up of the Harvard Growth Study of 1922 to 1935. N Engl J Med 1992;327:1350–5.

[32] Dietz WH. Health consequences of obesity in youth: childhood predictors of adult disease. Pediatrics 1998;101:518–25.

[33] Velasquez-Mieyer PA, Cowan PA, Cuervo R, et al. Does obesity matter in children with type 2 diabetes? Diabetes 2002;51:A362.

[34] Freedman DS, Bowman BA, Otvos JD, et al. Differences in the relation of obesity to serum triacylglycerol and VLDL subclass concentrations between black and white children: the Bogalusa Heart Study. Am J Clin Nutr 2002;75:827–33.

[35] Freedman DS, Dietz WH, Srinivasan SR, et al. The relation of overweight to cardiovascular risk factors among children and adolescents: the Bogalusa Heart Study. Pediatrics 1999;103: 1175–82.

[36] Freedman DS, Khan LK, Dietz WH, et al. Relationship of childhood obesity to coronary heart disease risk factors in adulthood: the Bogalusa Heart Study. Pediatrics 2001; 108:712–8.

[37] Frumkin H, editor. Environmental health: from global to local. San Francisco: John Wiley and Sons; 2005.

[38] Yanovski SZ, Yanovski JA. Obesity. N Engl J Med 2002;346:591–602.

[39] Wang G, Dietz WH. Economic burden of obesity in youths aged 6 to 17 years: 1979–1999. Pediatrics 2002;109:E81–E81.

[40] Powell LM, Slater S, Chaloupka FJ. The relationship between community physical activity settings and race, ethnicity, and socioeconomic status. Evidence-Based Prev Med 2004;1(2): 135–44.

[41] Burdette L, Whitaker RC. A national study of neighborhood safety, outdoor play, television viewing, and obesity in preschool children. Pediatrics 2005;116(3):657–62.

[42] Jones SE, Brener ND, McManus T. Prevalence of school policies, programs, and facilities that promote a healthy physical school environment. Am J Public Health 2003; 93(9):1570–5.

[43] US Government Accountability Office. School meal programs: competitive foods are widely available and generate substantial revenues for schools. Report no. GAO-05-563. US Government Accountability Office; 2005.

[44] Andrulis DP. Moving beyond the status quo in reducing racial and ethnic disparities in children's health. Public Health Rep 2005;12:370–7.

[45] Drewnowski A, Darmon N. The economics of obesity: dietary energy density and energy cost. Am J Clin Nutr 2005;82(1):S265–73.

[46] Grier SA, Brumbaugh AM. Noticing cultural differences: ad meanings created by target and non-target markets. J Advertising 1999;28:79–93.

[47] Holtzclaw B. Geographic Information System map: location of EJ communities to former PCB plant and other regulated facilities" using data at time of EPA Superfund intervention in 2000 namely: 2000 U.S. Census data; 2000 Housing Summary Tape File (STF3) data; EPA Region 4 environmental justice demographic thresholds for minority and low-income populations for Alabama; and 2000 Environmental Regulated Facility data; 2006.

[48] Bailey RK, Owens DL. Overcoming challenges in the diagnosis and treatment of attention-deficit/hyperactivity disorder in African Americans. J Natl Med Assoc 2005;97(10 Suppl): 5S–10S.

[49] Bussing R, Zima BT, Gary FA, et al. Barriers to detection, help-seeking, and service use for children with ADHD symptoms. J Behav Health Serv Res 2003;30:176–89.

[50] Canfield RL, Henderson CR Jr, Cory-Slechta DA, et al. Intellectual impairment in children with blood lead concentrations below 10 μg/dL. N Engl J Med 2003;248:1517–26.

[51] Chen A, Dietrich KN, Ware JH, et al. IQ and blood lead from 2 to 7 years – are the effects in older children the residual of high blood leads in 2 year olds? Environ Health Perspect 2005; 113(5):597–601.

[52] Koller K, Brown T, Spurgeon A, et al. Recent developments in low-level lead exposure and intellectual impairment in children. Environ Health Perspect 2004;112(9):987–94.

[53] Wood D. Effect of child and family poverty on child health in the United States. Pediatrics 2003;112:707–11.

[54] Shonkoff JP, Phillips DA, editors. From neurons to neighborhoods: the science of early childhood development. Institute of Medicine; Washington DC: National Academy Press, 2000. p. 274.

[55] Vision 2020 Organization. Vision 2020: for the Children of Anniston. Children's Health Environmental Justice Revitalization Project. Nomination and proposal for selection as an Interagency Working Group on Environmental Justice Demonstration Project. Anniston (AL): Vision 2020 Organization; 2002.

[56] Agency for Toxic Substances and Disease Registry. Toxicological profile for PCBs. Atlanta (GA): Agency for Toxic Substances and Disease Registry; 2000. p. 557–560.

[57] Canady R. Health consultation; evaluation of soil, blood, and air data from Anniston, Alabama. Atlanta (GA): Agency for Toxic Substances and Disease Registry; 2000.

[58] Kaplan S, Morris J. Kids at risk. US News World Rep 2000;128(24):47–53.

[59] Annie E. Casey Foundation. Kids count data book. Baltimore: Annie E. Casey Foundation; 1999

[60] Morrisey M, Stein J. for the Calhoun County Community Foundation. 2001 Health needs assessment: Calhoun County, Alabama. Birmingham (AL): University of Alabama at Birmingham; 2001.

[61] Massey D, Denton NA. American apartheid: segregation and the making of the underclass. Cambridge (MA): Harvard University Press; 1993.

[62] Bullard RD. People of color environmental groups: 2000 directory. Atlanta (GA): Environmental Justice Resource Center, Clark-Atlanta University; 2000. p. 1–21.

[63] Lee C. Environmental justice. In: Frumkin H, editor. Environmental health: from global to local. San Francisco: John Wiley and Sons; 2005.

[64] United Church of Christ Commission for Racial Justice. Toxic wastes and race in the United States: a national study on the racial and socio-economic characteristics of communities surrounding hazardous waste sites. New York: United Church of Christ; 1987.

[65] Lee C. Environmental justice: building a unified vision of health and environment. Environ Health Perspect 2002;110(Suppl 2):141–4.

[66] Executive Office of the President of the United States. Federal actions to address environmental justice in minority populations and low-income populations. Executive Order no. 12898. Fed Register 1994;59:7629.

[67] US Environmental Protection Agency, Office of Policy, Economics, and Innovation. Evaluating the use of partnerships to address environmental justice issues. EPA/100-R-03-001. Washington, DC: Environmental Protection Agency; 2003.

[68] Rodgers-Smith D, Holtzclaw B. A collaborative children's health project serving Anniston, AL. Presented at the National Community Involvement Conference. Philadelphia. July 23, 2003.

[69] Lasker RD, Weiss ES. Broadening participation in community problem solving: a multidisciplinary model to support collaborative practice and research. J Urban Health 2003;80: 14–57.

ELSEVIER
SAUNDERS

Pediatr Clin N Am
54 (2007) 399–415

PEDIATRIC CLINICS
OF NORTH AMERICA

Medical Laboratory Investigation of Children's Environmental Health

Harold E. Hoffman, MD, FRCPC, FACOEM[a],[*],
Ircna Buka, MBChB, FRCPC[b],[c],
Scott Phillips, MD, FACP, FACMT[d]

[a]*Department of Occupational Medicine, University of Alberta, 402 College Plaza,
8215-112 Street, Edmonton, Alberta T6G 2C8, Canada*
[b]*Department of Paediatrics, University of Alberta, 8213 Aberhart Centre,
11402 University Avenue NW, Edmonton, Alberta T6G 2C8, Canada*
[c]*Misericordia Community Hospital and Health Centre, 3 West Child Health Clinic,
16940-87th Avenue, Edmonton, Alberta T5R 4H5, Canada*
[d]*Division of Clinical Pharmacology & Toxicology, University of Colorado Health Sciences
Center, 10099 Ridge Gate Parkway, Suite 220, Lone Tree, CO 80124, USA*

Medical laboratory testing is an essential but very limited tool in the investigation and management of children with environmental chemical exposures and environmentally related disorders. Every day children are exposed to a wide variety of chemicals by breathing, eating, drinking, living, learning, and playing. Careful identification of potential exposures is essential before ordering tests. Quantifying environmental exposures in children requires understanding of the agent, the toxicology, the laboratory process, test capabilities, and test limitations. Although few exposures can be evaluated adequately by medical laboratory tests, exposure information can assist in the identification, prevention, or limiting of health problems. Medical laboratory tests may help the pediatrician understand exposures, health effects, diagnoses, causation, treatment, health risk, and prevention (Table 1).

Do children have different exposures?

The fetus is exposed to chemicals through the placenta. Teratogenic pharmaceuticals, such as thalidomide, demonstrate fetal vulnerabilities during the

---

* Corresponding author.
E-mail address: occmed@telus.net (H.E. Hoffman).

Table 1
Laboratory testing process

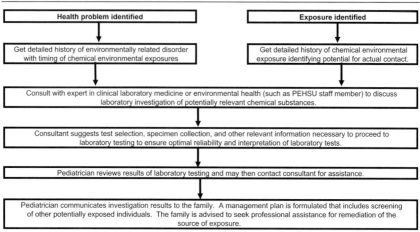

first 3 months of pregnancy when rapid growth and development of organs occurs. The fetus is susceptible to neurotoxins, such as lead and mercury [1].

After birth, newborns may face further environmental hazards. Breast milk may contain chemicals, such as polychlorinated biphenyls (PCBs) [1]. Water used to reconstitute formula may expose formula-fed infants to water contaminants. Dermal absorption in the newborn is increased because skin lacks adequate keratin for the first few days after birth. Newborns can develop hypothyroidism from iodine and betadine scrub solutions. Hexachlorophene can cause neurotoxicity in newborns [1].

As babies mature, solid foods are introduced, exposing them to pesticide residues in fruits, grains, and vegetables [1].

Children consume more calories per kilogram body weight and more milliliters of water per kilogram body weight than an adult. Therefore, the weight-adjusted dose of pollutants is more in children [1].

As children become mobile, their breathing zones are closer to the ground than that of an adult, making them more susceptible to the heavier chemicals that fall to the ground. At this stage, exposure vulnerability is increased by hand-to-mouth activity and ingestion of nonfood items. Young children's higher respiratory rate and increased minute ventilation make them more susceptible to inhalation exposure.

Children's increasing independence requires assessment of the environment of the home, day care, school, playground, or sports facility. In adolescent years, vocational training, employment, and risk-taking recreational activities expose adolescents to other hazards [1].

The child's socioeconomic status correlates with the child's susceptibility to exposures. Children of lower socioeconomic status are increasingly vulnerable to exposures through diet, play areas, school, housing, and residential location [1].

How can exposure be identified?

Identification of exposure is essential for selection of tests in the investigation of environmental health problems. Exposure is described by chemical type, route of exposure, and dose (Table 2). The route of exposure is the exposure pathway, such as inhalation, ingestion, or skin contact. Dose is the quantity, frequency, and duration of exposure.

To identify suspected chemical exposure, the pediatrician is encouraged to communicate with the patient, family, primary care physician, and laboratory expert. Exposure assessment requires inquiry about the child's residence regarding building type, plumbing (eg, lead pipes), flooring, heating system, age of construction, family home activities (hobbies), and proximity to facilities such as industrial plants. For example, in periurban communities in sub-Saharan Africa, children often live in homes with earthen floors or walls. These children have different exposures than children living in homes with carpeted or wood floors. Parental occupations may be relevant, because parents may bring home chemicals (eg, lead) on their clothes.

Outside the home, important activities of the child include school (building type and location relative to industry or high-voltage wires), child care facilities, travel to and from school, play activities, and family travel.

Table 2
Exposure factors used to characterize exposure

Characteristic	Explanation
Source	The source of exposure may identify the specific exposure, the distance from the source, the temperature, the wind direction, and frequency of release.
Type of exposure	Trade name, ingredients (components of the exposure)
Quantity of exposure	Dose (duration intermittent, prolonged)
Physical state	Gas, liquid, solid, dust, or vapor
Chemical characteristics	Reactivity, acid or base, explosive hazard, asphyxiate
Route of entry	Inhalation, ingestion, and dermal routes
Duration of exposure	The dose will be affected by the length of time of the exposure.
Frequency of exposure	Exposures may occur several times a day (eg, when children are exposed to smoking parents) or occasionally or rarely (eg, when children are exposed to lead when the parent melts lead for lead bullets or leaded glass).
Dates of exposure	The dates of exposure are important when evaluating test planning or test results. Exposure to carbon dioxide 2 days in the past cannot be measured, but long-term lead exposure occurring more than 2 days in the past can be measured.
Concurrent exposures	Exposures other than the primary exposure of concern may affect absorption, testing, or clinical findings. These other exposures also may be health hazards.

Because children may be employed, the child's occupational exposures must be described.

The pediatrician should ask about the type of exposure, the specific components of the exposure, the physical state (gas, liquid, solid, dust, vapor), route of exposure (inhalation, ingestion, dermal), duration, frequency, dates of exposure, and concurrent exposures.

Material Safety Data Sheets provide valuable basic product information, including

1. Product name, chemical name, and common names
2. Physical properties
3. Chemical characteristics
4. Physical hazards (flammability, explosion)
5. Health hazards
6. Routes of entry (inhalation, ingestion, skin contact, eye contact)
7. Exposure limits
8. Carcinogenic properties
9. Precautions for handling
10. Control measures
11. Emergency measures
12. Contact information for a responsible party

Material Safety Data Sheets are readily available at Vermont Safety Information Resources, Inc. (http://www2.hazard.com/index.php). They also are available from the manufacturer of the product in question.

The pediatrician is encouraged to collaborate with an industrial hygienist for exposure assessment and focused sampling. Industrial hygiene professionals evaluate exposures and exposure pathways in various media such as air, water, soil, and buildings. Industrial hygienists identify and measure exposures before they get to the child. Industrial hygienists traditionally focused on occupational settings, but they have become much more involved in environmental assessments in recent years. Industrial hygienists perform walk-through surveys to assess exposures. A walk-through survey is the first and most important technique to recognize health hazards [2]. Industrial hygienists quantify exposures by any potential route, such as air (inhalation), skin, and ingestion. Industrial hygienists can sample paint, soil, air, and water. Industrial hygienists have knowledge of the types of collecting equipment and the timing of sampling required to obtain valid and useful information.

What laboratory tests should be ordered when an exposure is identified?

When a child presents with a possible exposure, laboratory testing is not considered until a detailed exposure history and health history are taken and a physical examination is performed. Tests are used to confirm suspected exposures. Tests measure absorption by all routes, including inhalation, ingestion, and dermal routes.

Toxic chemicals in body fluids can be measured directly (measurements of metabolized chemical) or by indirect assessment (the effects on body systems). Measurements attempt to reflect the internal dose (body burden or amount of chemical in the child). Because the total amount of substance in the child cannot be measured, tests estimate the internal dose of the substance.

The pediatrician may communicate with a laboratory clinical consultant or environmental health expert (such as those at a Pediatric Environmental Health Specialty Unit [see the article by Davis and colleagues in this issue]) to discuss test selection, specimen collection, laboratory analysis, and interpretation. Before a test is ordered, the pediatrician should have some understanding of how to interpret the test.

In addition to levels of the chemical compound in the blood or the urine, specific end-organ effects (eg, liver or kidney damage in acute lead toxicity) must be assessed.

When one individual is thought to have been exposed to any substance, all potentially exposed people must be assessed. For example, when a child plays with liquid (elemental) mercury at school, laboratory tests can assess the child in a high-risk situation, but other children in the class must be tested also.

What difficulties are encountered with medical laboratory testing?

The chemical may be in a form that may not be accessible to laboratory testing. For example, lead is deposited in the bones and in the central nervous system, where lead concentrations cannot be measured readily [1].

Tests must be readily available. Although many compounds can be measured in research, the availability of routine medical laboratory testing for environmental chemicals is limited, and interpretation is difficult. Financial constraints limit the number of chemicals that can be tested.

The test collection must be convenient. Blood tests are painful for children, so alternate media, such as urine, may be considered. For children, 24-hour urine collection is difficult, so single-sample (spot) urine collections may be considered as an initial screen. If the spot urine test result is abnormal, a 24-hour urine sample is required to confirm the results of the spot urine test.

A routine clinical service laboratory offers a limited number of laboratory tests. Specimens often can be forwarded to a specialized laboratory to analyze other chemical compounds. Potentially hazardous levels for many substances cannot be provided because hazardous levels have not been established [3]. It is important to know the reliability of the laboratory before sending samples. Many laboratories purport to offer toxicologic evaluations of patient samples, but not all of these laboratories are reliable [4–6].

Planning may be required so that the collection facility and staff are ready for some tests. For example, special containers may need to be ordered. Specimen collection and processing may be difficult after usual laboratory work hours. The specimen may need to be collected at a specific time. End-of-shift collections may require laboratory staff to be available beyond their usual work hours. The timing of specimen collection after exposure depends on the duration of the agent or effect in the body (clearance rate). For example, trying to collect a carboxyhemoglobin (COHb) specimen early may be difficult. If COHb measurements for carbon monoxide exposure are not available urgently, COHb levels may have time to drop to zero, so the opportunity to confirm elevated carbon monoxide levels is missed. Collected samples may deteriorate overnight or undergo changes in the collection container. Collections may be difficult in remote situations.

Training of collection staff is required. Some specimen collections require unique procedures and equipment (eg, special containers) that require specific training of laboratory staff. Specimen collection must be performed carefully and accurately. The collection staff must know the correct collection container. Trace element–free containers must be used for trace element tests. The appropriate medium must be collected. Contamination must be avoided.

Processing, such as pipetting and centrifuging, must be done properly to avoid influence from other factors (eg, hemolysis, which releases high levels of elements in red blood cells).

The storage time from collection to testing may affect test results. Delay in testing may affect test results. Some tests not available locally require planning for administration (authorization and financial arrangements), collection time, collection containers, and transportation. Transportation of the specimen requires planning for collection, specimen safety, temperature maintenance, and laboratory acceptance of specimen. Transportation must be done promptly and with controlled temperature.

The time required to provide a laboratory report is important for clinical management. If results are not available for weeks, this information may not be useful to the pediatrician's management of the case. Promptness of laboratory testing (turnaround time) is important; some laboratories test batches (20–40 samples), so testing is delayed until enough samples are received.

What can the pediatrician do to ensure good specimen collection?

Because most substances are excreted over time, delay in testing limits the ability to measure peak levels of the substance. Volatile agents are excreted quickly, so testing must be done immediately after exposure. Substances with short half-lives in the body, such as carbon monoxide, require measurement immediately after exposure. In most cases, tests done months or years after exposure are not useful. For arsenic tests, no seafood should be eaten for 3 days before testing, because seafood contains organic arsenic. Organic arsenic is not toxic but may contribute to the total arsenic levels.

The pediatrician should select the best collection media (urine or blood) for each chemical. The laboratory clinical consultant can provide this information.

To obtain serum, blood is collected without anticoagulant, is allowed to clot, is centrifuged, and the supernatant is collected. Serum is useful for substances that are dissolved in blood or bound to serum proteins.

To obtain plasma, blood is collected with an anticoagulant and centrifuged to collect supernatant.

Whole blood is collected with an anticoagulant. Whole blood is preferred for testing of substances that exist primarily in red cells.

Urine tests measure excretion. Renal excretion is related to systemic disease, hydration, and exposures. Aluminum, arsenic, cadmium, copper, mercury, and selenium can be measured in the urine. A single urine sample is not as accurate as a 24-hour collection.

How can the pediatrician identify a good laboratory?

Selection of a laboratory for testing depends on factors including turnaround time (measured from test ordering to result receipt), accuracy of results, test menu, accreditation, availability of staff to consult with the ordering physician, and test cost. Medical laboratories must have reliable processing and quality control, certification, and efficient reporting of results. The accuracy of results can be assessed by reviewing 1 to 2 years of graded proficiency specimen testing results (unknown specimens submitted by a regulatory or accrediting organization). To review the proficiency results critically, these results can be examined for the presence of significant analytical trends as well as near misses [7]. All laboratories in the United States (including research laboratories) that perform diagnostic testing on human material must have government certification. For Clinical Laboratory Improvement Amendments certification, trace element laboratories must comply with regulations for proficiency testing, quality control, quality assurance, patient test management, personnel, certification, and inspections [8]. Because the Clinical Laboratory Improvement Amendments certification is the minimum requirement for laboratory operation, many laboratories have sought additional accreditation from laboratory professional accrediting organizations such as the College of American Pathologists [9]. If the pediatrician has difficulty confirming the accreditation status of a laboratory, the laboratory, a toxicologist, or an occupational medicine specialist can be consulted.

Research laboratories may measure chemicals that are specific for particular research scenarios. Research laboratories might not be accredited to perform clinical tests. Clinical tests require ongoing quality control and formal accreditation.

What should a pediatrician do after diagnosing a condition that might be caused by an environmental exposure?

An increasing number of childhood conditions are being recognized as having an environmental link. Parents often ask why their child has specific symptoms, such as sleep disturbance, headaches, growth failure, and diseases such as asthma, cancer, and neurodevelopmental disorders. Taking a detailed exposure history in these circumstances is paramount to offering a satisfactory response. Because of the long latency periods between exposure and identification of clinical effects, it often is difficult to confirm the etiology of the presenting, possibly environmentally related, disorder. An increasing number of common childhood conditions may have an environmental link identified only on careful exposure history taking and supporting laboratory evidence. Examples are failure to thrive or iron-deficiency anemia linked to lead exposure [10]. A further example could be a child who has recurrent headaches that occur particularly in the morning linked to carbon monoxide exposure. In both circumstances, the results of laboratory testing may be normal unless performed soon after exposure.

To confirm that a substance caused the health condition, the following concepts must be considered [11]:

- Define the health condition specifically and confirm that the child really has the condition of concern. For example, after carbon monoxide exposure, cognition problems could be caused by both carbon monoxide exposure and secondary psychologic issues. Neuropsychologic testing is required to confirm that a neurocognitive problem exists.
- Is the substance known in the scientific literature to cause the condition? For example, many health problems may be reported after an exposure. The pediatrician should review the literature to determine which problems are known to result from a specific exposure.
- What is the weight of the scientific evidence? What are the relative risk or odds ratios? For example, a child living near high-voltage wires may develop leukemia. A pediatrician could determine if there might be a relationship between the exposure and the outcome by reviewing the literature for information on relative risk or odds ratios between exposed and nonexposed children.
- Temporality: Did exposure precede the health condition with appropriate latency? Latency is the time delay between exposure and health effect. For example, carbon monoxide and organophosphate pesticides may have an immediate effect. Lead effects may take a much longer time to be identified clinically. Exposure of children to asbestos may cause asbestos pulmonary fibrosis and cancers that may not be detectable for decades [12]. To account for latency, tests should be done at intervals relevant to the exposure. For example, six children in an elementary school developed leukemia, but investigation revealed that the children had started this school only 1 or 2 months previously. The leukemia was subclinical for several months, so the new school exposure did not precede the onset of leukemia. Also, the latency period from exposure to leukemia development would be a couple of years. These temporality issues determined that the new school did not cause the leukemias.

- Was the internal dose (amount of substance reaching the affected organ) sufficient to cause the condition? Was the internal dose above the threshold of effect for the substance? Answering these questions requires estimation of peak dose after exposure. For example, with carbon monoxide exposure, the highest carboxyhemoglobin level correlates with peak internal dose and potential for adverse health effects.
- Are other exposed individuals affected? People other than the index case (initial case identified) may have confirmed exposures or identified similar health effects from this exposure. Similarly exposed individuals provide supportive evidence that the exposure was hazardous.
- Do measurements correlate with toxicity? The identified blood or urine levels must be in a range known to cause toxicity.
- Did other (concurrent) exposures occur? Were health effects or measured medical test levels caused by an identified exposure or by other (concurrent) exposures? One must consider other causes of the health problem, including other exposures, medications, or concurrent health conditions.

If a clinical picture suggests an exposure syndrome, a pediatrician may wish to pursue laboratory testing. For example, when a child presents with headache, carbon monoxide exposure should be considered in the differential diagnosis. Carbon monoxide–induced headaches may be suspected when a child experiences morning headaches after sleeping in a basement bedroom near a furnace. A qualified professional can measure the carbon monoxide level in the air in the home. A carboxyhemoglobin level may be measured in the symptomatic child, although carboxyhemoglobin levels decrease rapidly once the child is removed from the exposure.

In the case of a neurodevelopmental disorder, it is important to pursue an exposure history. The exposure history looks for possible exposures to neurotoxicants, such as lead, mercury, or PCBs, that may have occurred several years previously. Laboratory testing of the chemical compounds in the body may fail to confirm the diagnosis if the child was removed from the source of exposure several months previously. Growth failure, recurrent abdominal pain, and sleep problems may result from lead exposure, and a serum lead needs to be considered in these children.

Is there a need to assess apparently healthy children for exposures?

Populations of children can be tested to determine levels of substances of concern. Exposure trends (increasing or decreasing levels in children) may be found. Children who require further assessment or treatment can be identified.

Children can be tested in the following ways:

- Screening is a one-time event that looks for the early effects of hazards. In screening, populations are tested to identify children who may be helped by further testing or treatment to reduce the risk of health problems.

- Surveillance involves the regular examination of people who are at risk for disease. Tests are done to detect changes before health problems occur [13]. Surveillance is the ongoing, systematic collection, analysis, interpretation, and dissemination of data regarding a health-related event [14,15].
- Targeted testing is performed on children with possible higher exposures.

What is the risk of a health problem from an exposure?

Risk is the possibility of suffering a harmful event. Risk is the chance that a health problem will occur following an exposure. Risk factors are associated with increased chance of getting a specific disease. The internal dose of a chemical is the primary determinant of risk.

The child's risk of toxicity may be assessed directly through specimen levels (eg, lead, mercury, arsenic) [1]. Laboratory testing for organophosphate pesticide poisoning uses indirect methods by measuring levels of acetylcholinesterase, a neurotransmitter that accumulates when organophosphate pesticide exposure is significant [1].

Phases of individual risk assessment may include the following [13]:

1. Hazard identification is used to determine whether exposure to an agent can produce a health problem.
2. Exposure estimation involves measuring the intensity, frequency, and duration of exposures to an agent.
3. Dose–response assessment relates the dose of an agent received to the incidence of an adverse health effect.
4. Risk characterization is an estimate of the incidence of an adverse health effect under the conditions of exposure.

The pediatrician should be aware of emerging science regarding identified adverse health effects at lower levels of exposure (Fig. 1).

In children a blood lead level of more than 60 μg/dL is a medical emergency, because these children may develop encephalopathy resulting in stupor, seizures, and coma. Lower blood lead levels may be associated with anemia, abdominal pain, constipation, headaches, and agitation.

Pediatricians are increasingly concerned that certain substances have no threshold for safety. Chronic blood lead concentrations, even below 10 μg/dL, are associated with decrease in children's intelligence scores [7]. Currently, regulatory levels in the United States and Canada are still set at 10 μg/dL [10]. There is sufficient and compelling scientific evidence to lower the blood level action level to 2 μg/dL [16].

Carbon monoxide intoxication can cause headaches at lower levels of exposure and convulsions, coma, and death at higher levels (Table 3) [1].

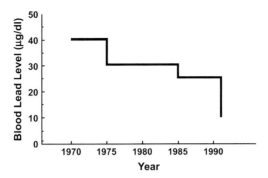

Fig. 1. Blood lead levels considered elevated by the Centers for Disease Control and the Public Health Service. (*Courtesy of* the US Department of Health and Human Services, Public Health Service, Centers for Disease Control. Preventing lead poisoning in young children. Publication date: 10/01/1991. Available at: http://wonder.cdc.gov/wonder/prevguid/p0000029/p0000029. asp#Figure_2_2). Accessed March 1, 2007.

What unusual specialized tests can be done?

Tests on unusual specimens are rarely useful in clinical practice. For example, manganese and zinc are often measured, but interpretation is difficult. No relation exists between manganese concentration in urine or blood and severity of chronic manganese poisoning. No safe level has been identified. When children are exposed to high levels of manganese or zinc, the urine and blood levels will be quite variable. Higher exposures do not correlate with high manganese or zinc levels in the urine or blood.

Hair and nail tests have no clinical applicability. For most substances, insufficient data currently exist to allow the prediction of a health effect from the concentration of the substance in hair [17]. Although methylmercury can be tested in hair, this testing is primarily a research procedure. For hair and nail testing, potential external contamination (shampoo, airborne substance) prevents interpretation of results.

Table 3
Risk of carbon monoxide health effects is related to blood carboxyhemoglobin

Blood carboxyhemoglobin (%)	Possible health effects
< 1	No effects
5–10	Visual disturbances
10–30	Headaches
40–50	Fainting and collapse
50–60	Coma and convulsions
60–80	Possible death

Data from Workplace Health and Safety, Government of Alberta. Work Safe Alberta: Carbon monoxide at the work site. Available at: http://employment.alberta.ca/whs/network/hstopics/chemical/co.asp. Accessed March 1, 2007.

Breast milk, cord blood, and fat biopsies are not readily available. Breast milk is not tested in clinical situations. Breast milk has been used extensively in research regarding environmental exposures.

For serum or adipose tissue PCB levels, clinical interpretation is difficult [18]. PCB tests are likely to be inconclusive, so analysis of serum or adipose tissue samples is not recommended unless the exposure has been massive [18].

How should test results be interpreted?

The physician should plan in advance for the interpretation by identifying the best test and the test result ranges that are clinically significant (eg, the toxic range). A test should not be ordered unless the physician knows what to do with the result.

For many chemicals, it is not known how to apply the measurements clinically [3]. Consultation with a knowledgeable expert, such as a toxicologist or occupational medicine specialist, may be considered at the test selection phase (Table 4).

The ability to measure something does not mean that measurement should be done. For example, in industrial settings, exposure to aluminum can cause toxicity, but plasma and urine aluminum levels do not reflect respiratory or neurologic toxicity [19]. Urine aluminum is a more sensitive indicator of aluminum exposure than serum aluminum, but the half-life in urine (and blood) is very short [20]. Accurate levels for concern (biologic

Table 4
Examples of available tests

Exposure	Best specimen for analysis	Accuracy	Factors affecting measured levels	Level of concern for health in a child
Arsenic	24-hour urine		Seafood ingested within 3 days before testing.	Because no threshold is present, no safe level is identified.
Carbon monoxide	Blood		Cigarette smoking	Carboxyhemoglobin 8%, but levels may be higher in smokers.
Lead	Blood	Very accurate		Blood 0.48 μmol/L = 10 μg/dL Because no threshold is present, no safe level is identified.
Mercury	24-hour urine; blood is alternate specimen		Fish consumption, dental amalgam fillings, alcohol consumption	Because no threshold is present, safe levels are difficult to define.

threshold values) are not available. Science has not yet identified the aluminum levels at which no health problems can occur.

Laboratory results must be interpreted in relation to clinical information. Interpretation requires a comprehensive pediatric assessment that includes medical documents, medical history, exposure history, physical examination, imaging, and laboratory investigations. Interpretation requires understanding of the clinical situation, the agent (physical properties, kinetics, metabolism, excretion, and toxicity), test selection, test timing, collection factors, and internal laboratory factors. Usually, limited information is available regarding exposure, concurrent exposures, health problems, and medications. The physician must extrapolate from available information.

Interpretation requires attention to the many different units of measure that are used. Potential for error exists when translating different units. Some units are difficult to compare, such as units/gram creatinine to units/liter.

Interpretation is more accurate if clinical information and other laboratory tests support the findings of an elevated level. Abnormal liver function tests or abnormal kidney function tests may provide supportive evidence of exposure in relation to a substance that is known to be hepatotoxic or nephrotoxic. If test results are not consistent with clinical information or other tests, the pediatrician should review the whole case and investigation.

Reference ranges usually represent the concentrations in a normal population. If health surveillance has not been done, the reference range may not represent the test values in the population of concern. The range at which toxicity is expected may be much higher than the reference range. Laboratories set their own reference ranges, so reference ranges vary between laboratories (Table 5).

Government agencies often provide regulations for blood or urine measurements (action levels). When the individual has levels above the regulatory level, some action is required, such as removal from exposure. Regulatory standards generally apply only to adults, not children. Regulatory exposure levels do not guarantee that every child is safe at these levels. Regulatory levels are influenced by science (toxicology and risk assessment), politics, and economics. The process of altering regulatory reference ranges appropriately according to available science is lengthy and depends on many factors, including the methods available for risk assessment [21]. The pediatrician who interprets the tests should not merely refer to the regulatory reference range but should consider emerging science [16].

For some chemicals, a long period of time passes before the toxic effects become apparent. Delayed neurologic sequelae from carbon monoxide may not be apparent for weeks (from 3–240 days), long after the several hours required for carbon monoxide to returned to pre-exposure levels [1]. Latency is the time period between the exposure event and clinical evidence of a disease process. A long latency period may allow time for the test to

Table 5
Definitions of laboratory result references

Laboratory result	Definition
Laboratory detection limit	Lowest amount measurable. Detection limit should be specified for each laboratory report. Accuracy of measurement declines as detection limit is approached. Laboratory results that are near the detection limit are an accuracy concern
Normal range	Range of 95% of healthy subjects. Upper and lower limits are based on 2 SDs from the mean. Values outside this range are considered abnormal, although these values will occur in 5% of healthy people. Normal ranges are derived from healthy people. This normal range has no relationship to the toxic threshold of the substance.
Population reference range	The population reference range indicates the test value expected from usual exposure in daily life (background level in population). Laboratory reports usually indicate population reference range rather than levels of concern or toxic range. Reference ranges are derived from sampling of individuals considered representative of the whole population. Convenient people (convenience sample) are the usual source of data for reference ranges. A local population may be different from the population used for reference. Reference ranges are usually derived from a small convenience sample, population samples, published studies, the laboratory's experience, other laboratories, or expedient ranges (to give reasonable numbers of positives and negatives.). Reference ranges are inconsistent between laboratories. The source of reference ranges for individual laboratories usually is not readily available. Most laboratories do not have reference ranges for children. Reference ranges do not account for vulnerability factors, such as age, size, reproduction (adolescents), concurrent illness, medications, and concurrent exposures.
Biologic exposure indices	The concentration below which nearly all people should not experience adverse health effects. Biologic exposure indices usually are written for young healthy adult males, not for women, children, or vulnerable people. Safe levels are often determined from both toxicologic and administrative factors.
Toxic threshold	Lowest level at which adverse health effects are expected. Toxicity thresholds vary with individual factors, exposure dose, and exposure rate. Toxicity thresholds are often orders of magnitude greater than the reference ranges.

return to normal before clinical effects become apparent. The damage has been done, and the chemical has been excreted or stored (eg, lead is stored in bone). In neurodevelopment cases, toxicity may have occurred a long time before the problem is identified, so measurements of chemicals might be normal. For example, by the time that lead-induced neurodevelopmental problems are identified, the lead levels may decrease to a lower (normal)

Table 6
Follow-up testing of children with elevated blood lead levels

Initial test (µg/dL)	Follow-up test
10–19	3 months
20–44	1 month – 1 week[a]
45–59	48 hours
60–69	24 hours
70 or higher	Immediately as an emergency test

[a] The higher the screening blood lead level, the more urgent is the need for a diagnostic test.
From: the Centers for Disease Control and Prevention., Screening young children for lead poisoning: guidance for state and local public health officials. In: Roles of child health-care providers in childhood lead poisoning prevention. November 1997. Available at: http://www.cdc.gov/nceh/lead/guide/1997/pdf/chapter4.pdf. Accessed March 1, 2007.

range [1]. Interpretation may be limited by a long latency period between exposure and clinical effect.

What should the pediatrician do after laboratory tests confirm an exposure?

After exposure is identified, the child and other potentially exposed people must be removed from further exposure. Decontamination may be required. Health problems must be treated. Elevated chemicals in the body may require specific treatment. Adequate long-term follow-up, such as neurodevelopmental testing for children with carbon monoxide or lead exposure, or chest radiographs for those with asbestos exposure, are also important (Table 6) [10].

Summary

Medical laboratory testing is vital for investigating and managing children who have environmentally related disorders and children with environmental chemical exposures. Few of these compounds can be measured in a routine clinical service laboratory. An understanding of the exposure circumstances and toxicology of the agent is required for the ordering and interpretation of tests.

Many limitations exist regarding test selections, specimen collection, laboratory analysis, and interpretation. A detailed clinical history as well as any potential chemical exposures needs to be elicited by the physician and shared with the laboratory expert. This consultation allows better accuracy in test selection, specimen collection, and interpretation of results and should take place before any laboratory tests are ordered. Test interpretation requires understanding of the capabilities and limitations of these tests.

Adequate investigation, management, and follow-up of exposed children are mandatory.

Acknowledgments

Dr. George Cembrowski, Director, Medical Biochemistry, Laboratory Medicine and Pathology, University of Alberta Hospital, Edmonton, Alberta, contributed to the information on laboratory selection.

Further reading

Advisory Committee on Childhood Lead Poisoning Prevention. Recommendations for blood lead screening of young children enrolled in Medicaid: targeting a group at high risk. MMWR Morb Mortal Wkly Rep 2002;49:1–13 Available at: http://www.cdc.gov/mmwr/PDF/RR/RR4914.pdf. Accessed March 1, 2007.
Centers for Disease Control and Prevention (CDC). Roles of child health-care providers in childhood lead poisoning prevention. In: Screening young children for lead poisoning: guidance for state and local public health officials. Atlanta (GA): Centers for Disease Control and Prevention; 1997. Available at: http://www.cdc.gov/nceh/lead/guide/1997/pdf/chapter4.pdf. Accessed March 1, 2007.
Commission for Environmental Cooperation. Children's health and the environment in North America: a first report on available indicators and measures. 2006. Available at: http://www.cec.org/files/pdf/POLLUTANTS/CEH-Indicators-fin_en.pdf. Accessed March 1, 2007.
Greenberg MI, editor-in-Chief. Occupational, industrial, and environmental toxicology. 2nd edition. Philadelphia: Mosby; p. 312–25.
Guidotti T, Audette R, Martin C. Interpretation of trace metal analysis profile for patients occupationally exposed to metals. Occup Med (Lond) 1997;47:497–503.
Levy BS, Wegman DH. Occupational health recognizing and preventing work-related disease. 3rd edition. New York: Little, Brown and Company; 1995. p. 285.
Third National Report on Human Exposure to Environmental Chemicals. NCEH publication # 05-0570. p. 1–475. Atlanta (GA); NCEH; 2005. Available at: http://www.cdc.gov/exposurereport/3rd/pdf/thirdreport.pdf. Accessed March 1, 2007.
US Department of Health and Human Services, Public Health Service, Centers for Disease Control. Preventing lead poisoning in young children. Available at: http://wonder.cdc.gov/wonder/prevguid/p0000029/p0000029.asp#Figure_2_2. Accessed October 1, 1991.
Varon J, Marik PE. Carbon monoxide poisoning. The Internet Journal of Emergency and Intensive Care Medicine 1997;1(2). Available at: http://www.ispub.com/ostia/index.php?xmlFilePath=journals/ijeicm/vol1n2/CO.xml. Accessed March 1, 2007.
Work Safe Alberta: Workplace Health and Safety Bulletin. Carbon monoxide at the work site Table 1: Health effects and COHb levels from acute exposure to carbon monoxide. Alberta Workplace Health and Safety. 2003–2004. Available at: http://www3.gov.ab.ca/hre/whs/publications/pdf/ch031.pdf. Accessed March 1, 2007.

References

[1] American Academy of Pediatrics Committee on Environmental Health. Lead. In: Etzel RA, editor. Pediatric environmental health. 2nd edition. Elk Grove Village (IL): American Academy of Pediatrics; 2003. p. 249–66.
[2] LaDou J. Current occupational & environmental medicine. In: Fowler DP, editor. Industrial hygiene. 3rd edition. New York: Lange Medical Books; 2004. p. 638–54.
[3] Centers for Disease Control and Prevention. Department of Health and Human Services. Third national report on human exposure to environmental chemicals. NCEH publication #05-0570. Atlanta (GA): Centers for Disease Control and Prevention; 2005. p. 1–475. Available at: http://www.cdc.gov/exposurereport/3rd/pdf/thirdreport.pdf. Accessed March 1, 2007.

[4] Seidel S, Kreutzer R, Smith D, et al. Assessment of commercial laboratories performing hair mineral analysis. JAMA 2001;285(1):67–72.

[5] Harkins DK, Susten AS. Hair analysis: exploring the state of the science. Environ Health Perspect 2003;111(4):576–8.

[6] Barrett S. Commercial hair analysis. Science or scam? JAMA 1985;254(8):1041–5.

[7] Carey RN, Cembrowski GS, Garber CC, et al. Performance characteristics of several rules for self-interpretation of proficiency testing data. Arch Pathol Lab Med 2005;129:997–1003.

[8] US Department of Health and Human Services, Health Care Financing Administration, Public Health Service, Medicare, Medicaid and Clinical Laboratory Improvement Amendments programs. Regulations implementing the Clinical Laboratory Improvement Amendments of 1988. Federal Register, February 28, 1992;57:7002–243.

[9] College of American Pathologists. Available at: www.cap.org.

[10] Tsekrekos S, Buka I. Lead levels in Canadian children: do we have to review the standard? J Paediatr Child Health 2005;10(4):215–20.

[11] Hill AB. The environment and disease: association or causation. Proc R Soc Med 1965;58: 295–300.

[12] Miller A. Mesothelioma in household members of asbestos-exposed workers: 32 United States cases since 1990. Am J Ind Med 2005;47(5):458–62.

[13] Hoffman HE, Guidotti TL. Basic clinical skills in occupational medicine. Prim Care 1994; 21(7):225–36.

[14] Centers for Disease Control and Prevention, Department of Health and Human Services. Statistics and surveillance. Available at: http://www.cdc.gov/hiv/topics/surveillance/print/index.htm. Accessed March 1, 2007.

[15] Canfield RL, Henderson CR, Cory-Slechta DA, et al. Intellectual impairment in children with blood lead concentrations below 10 µg per deciliter. N Engl J Med 2003;348(16): 1517–26.

[16] Gilbert SG, Weiss B. A rationale for lowering the blood lead action level from 10 to 2 µg/dL. Neurotoxicology 2006;27(5):693–701. Available at: http://www.sciencedirect.com.

[17] Agency for Toxic Substances and Disease Registry. Hair Analysis Panel Discussion. Summary report: hair analysis panel discussion: exploring the state of the science. June 12–13, 2001. Prepared for: The Agency for Toxic Substances and Disease Registry (ATSDR) Division of Health Assessment and Consultation and Division of Health Education and Promotion, Atlanta, GA,. by Eastern Research Group, 110 Hartwell Avenue, Lexington, MA 02421. December 2001. Page VII. Available at: http://www.atsdr.cdc.gov/HAC/hair_analysis/hairanalysis.pdf. Accessed March 1, 2007.

[18] Agency for Toxic Substances and Disease Registry. Polychlorinated (PCB) Toxicity Laboratory Tests Available at: http://www.atsdr.cdc.gov/HEC/CSEM/pcb/lab_tests.html. Accessed March 1, 2007.

[19] Rosenstock L, Cullen MR, Brodkin CA, et al. Textbook of clinical occupational and environmental medicine. 2nd edition. New York: Elsevier Saunders; 2005. p. 943–5.

[20] Wilhelm M, Ewers U, Schulz C. Revised and new reference values for some trace elements in blood and urine for human biomonitoring in environmental medicine. Int J Hyg Environ Health 2004;207:69–73.

[21] Environmental Protection Agency. Risk assessment guidelines. Available at: http://www.epa.gov/ncea/raf/rafguid.htm. Accessed March 1, 2007.

ELSEVIER
SAUNDERS

Pediatr Clin N Am
54 (2007) 417–424

PEDIATRIC CLINICS
OF NORTH AMERICA

Index

Note: Page numbers of article titles are in **boldface** type.

A

Acrodynia, 243

Adoptees, international, lead levels in, 274

Aeroallergens
climate change and, 219–220
in home environment, 298

Air pollution
indoor. *See* Air quality, indoor.
outdoor, 345–347
climate change and, 219–220
environmental health disparities in, 382–383

Air purifiers, 299

Air quality
indoor, **295–307**
global view of, 345–347
health effects of, 346–347
improvement of, 304–305
in home environment, 295–301
in occupational environment, 303–304
in play environment, 302–303
in school environment, 301–302
mycotoxins and, 318–320
outdoor. *See* Air pollution, outdoor.

Alimentary toxic aleukia, 318

Allergens
in home environment, 298
mold as, 310–318
outdoor, climate change and, 219–220

Allergic bronchopulmonary mycosis, 312, 315

Allergic fungal sinusitis, 312, 315–316

Allergic rhinitis, mold-induced, 312, 314–315

Alternaria, health effects of, 311, 314, 317–318

Alternative remedies, lead in, 274–276

Amalgams, dental, mercury exposure from, 253–257

Anniston, Alabama, industrial pollution in, community action for, 386–392

Arsenic poisoning, 341, 410

Arts and crafts supplies, chemical hazards in, 357

Asbestos exposure, in school renovation, 356

Aspergillus, health effects of, 311, 315–318, 321

Asphalt fumes, in school environment, 356

Asthma
air pollution and, 345–346
environmental health disparities in, 382–383
in smoke exposure, 296
mold-induced, 311–312, 314

Atopic dermatitis, mold-induced, 315

Attention-deficit hyperactivity disorder, environmental health disparities in, 385–386

Autism
mercury exposure and, 251–253
pica behavior in, lead exposure and, 273–274

B

BAL (dimercaprol)
for lead exposure, 286
for mercury exposure, 251

Baseball, injuries in, 363–365

Bipolaris, health effects of, 315–316

Boletus edulis, health effects of, 315

Breast milk
lead in, 276
mercury in, 255–257

British anti-Lewisite (dimercaprol)
for lead exposure, 286
for mercury exposure, 251

Bronchiolitis, in smoke exposure, 297

Moving?

Make sure your subscription moves with you!

To notify us of your new address, find your **Clinics Account Number** (located on your mailing label above your name), and contact customer service at:

E-mail: elspcs@elsevier.com

800-654-2452 (subscribers in the U.S. & Canada)
407-345-4000 (subscribers outside of the U.S. & Canada)

Fax number: 407-363-9661

Elsevier Periodicals Customer Service
6277 Sea Harbor Drive
Orlando, FL 32887-4800

*To ensure uninterrupted delivery of your subscription, please notify us at least 4 weeks in advance of move.

ELSEVIER